AF507858

"Dreameaz: A System for People Who Have Tried Everything and Still Can't Sleep"

By Paul Szyarto

Copyright © 2026 Paul Szyarto
All rights reserved.

No part of this book may be reproduced, stored in a retrieval system, or transmitted in any form or by any means, electronic, mechanical, photocopying, recording, or otherwise, without the prior written permission of the publisher, except for brief quotations in reviews.

Published by **PSG Publishing**
United States of America

ISBN (Paperback): 979-8-9944789-0-5

This book is intended for informational and educational purposes only. It is not medical advice and should not be used as a substitute for professional diagnosis or treatment. Always consult a qualified healthcare provider regarding any questions you may have about sleep, health conditions, medications, or treatments.

The author and publisher disclaim any liability arising directly or indirectly from the use or application of the information contained in this book.

First Edition
Printed in the United States of America

For those who struggle with sleep.

**Every sleepless night has a cause.
We'll help you find yours.**

You don't need to read this book in order.
You don't need to try everything at once.
And you don't need to believe that sleep is something you've
lost forever.

This isn't about forcing sleep or chasing perfect nights.
It's about understanding what's quietly getting in the way,
and removing it.

Take this at your own pace.
Read what resonates.
Skip what doesn't.

Sleep returns when the conditions are right.

Introduction: The Night I Reached My Breaking Point

There's a moment in every person's life when the world finally becomes quiet enough for the truth to slip through. For me, it happened on a night that looked completely ordinary from the outside, no crisis, no drama, nothing that should have set it apart. But sometimes the nights that look the calmest are the ones that expose how much noise you've been carrying inside.

I remember lying there in the dark, staring at the ceiling long after the house had gone still. My body felt heavy, but my mind was pacing like it had somewhere urgent to be. Thoughts looped without direction. My heartbeat felt louder than it should. My chest was tight, not painful, but braced, as if I were preparing for something I couldn't name. I wasn't in danger, yet my mind behaved like it was waiting for impact.

There wasn't one problem keeping me awake. No trauma replaying itself. No crisis demanding attention. It was something far more subtle, and in its own way, far more frightening:

I had lost the ability to shut down.

Not suddenly. Sleep rarely disappears in a single moment. It slips away gradually. A few restless nights. A couple of early mornings. A little anxiety as you try to drift off. That familiar sense of dread as the sun goes down because you know what's coming.

And then one day you look back and realize you can't remember the last time sleep felt natural, easy, or restorative.

That night, as I lay awake long after exhaustion should have taken over, I felt the weight of years pressing down on me, years of pushing too hard, working too long, carrying too much. Layers of stress I never paused long enough to peel back. Years of telling myself I was fine, that I just needed to push a little harder, that people like me don't get the luxury of falling apart.

But the truth is simple:

Pushing through stops working the moment your nervous system stops listening.

And that was exactly what was happening.

All the discipline, grit, and mental toughness I'd built over a lifetime weren't helping me here. If anything, they made things worse. I tried to "power down," to force my mind into stillness, to control my way into sleep the same way I controlled everything else.

But sleep doesn't respond to force.

It responds to alignment.

I didn't know that then. All I knew was that I was losing a battle I didn't understand. And that scared me in a way I wasn't used to. Not because I feared sleeplessness itself, but because of what it revealed, the state of my body, my mind, my identity.

When you build your entire sense of self on being strong, capable, and in control, realizing your basic functioning is slipping feels like an internal betrayal.

That was when everything caught up with me.

The sleeplessness wasn't the enemy; it was the signal. My body's final warning that I'd been operating past my limits for too long. I had mistaken endurance for health. I had confused resilience with avoidance. I ignored the signs until they grew too loud to silence.

And in that dark room, I finally understood something that would change the course of my life:

Willpower can carry you through almost anything… except the moments when your physiology refuses to follow.

Most people never hear that truth. I certainly didn't, not until it was too late.

This book exists so you don't have to wait for your own breaking point. You deserve a guide who isn't speaking from theory, but from lived experience. Someone who understands that sleep loss is not an inconvenience, it is a slow erosion of identity, patience, health, and your ability to function in the world.

There are plenty of books written by experts who study sleep professionally. This isn't one of them.

This is a book written by someone who lived the consequences of broken sleep, physically, emotionally, biologically, and had to rebuild himself from the inside out. Someone who had to uncover the real reasons sleep fails. Someone who couldn't afford generic advice that wasn't built for real lives and real stress.

You won't find "hacks" in these pages. You won't find quick fixes that crumble the moment life gets hard.

This book is built on two things:

1. Lived Experience
Years of wrestling with a body that refused to shut down.
Years of tracing symptoms back to their roots, behavioral, biological, emotional.
Years of learning what actually works in the real world.

2. A Proven Method
The Dreameaz Method™, born from experience, refined through research, and tested with real users. A method designed for those who feel like sleep is no longer possible.

This book is for:

- the person who wakes at 3 AM and can't shut their mind off

- the person who feels like their body is betraying them

- the person who has tried everything and still can't sleep

- the high-functioning individual who's unraveling on the inside

- the person who doesn't want to rely on medication forever

- the person desperate for clarity, calm, and restoration

And it's also for the person who hasn't hit their breaking point yet, but feels themselves moving toward it.

If your nights feel long, your days feel foggy, and your mind won't quiet down no matter how tired you are, you're in the right place.

This is the book I wish someone had handed me before my life fell apart.

And it's the one I'm honored to place in your hands now. Because no matter how long it's been, no matter how deep the struggle feels, no matter how many nights you've spent hoping things would change…

You can sleep again.

Your body remembers how.
Your mind remembers how.
And together, we're going to bring you back to that place, naturally, powerfully, permanently.

Chapter 1: The Silent Collapse: What Happens When You Stop Sleeping

Section 1: The Slow Breakdown You Don't Notice Until It's Too Late

Sleep doesn't fail dramatically.

It fades. Almost politely at first.

You don't wake up one morning and suddenly discover your ability to sleep has disappeared. It unravels slowly, subtle enough to dismiss, quiet enough to excuse, and gradual enough to label as "just a busy week" or "just a little stress." That's the cruelty of broken sleep: it gives you just enough performance to believe everything is fine, right up until the moment it isn't.

The breakdown starts with small changes you barely notice:

- You take a few minutes longer to fall asleep.

- Your mind feels slightly more active at night.

- You wake once or twice but fall back asleep quickly.

- You chalk it up to a late coffee or a long day.

Then the pattern shifts.

It becomes harder to settle in.
Your body feels wired when it's supposed to be winding down.
You wake earlier than you want to but tell yourself you'll "catch up" on the weekend.
You push through the day because that's what you've always done.

Eventually, the nights feel different.
Not terrible, just… off.

You lie down tired, but you don't drift.
Your thoughts loop in ways they didn't before.
The room is the same, but your mind behaves like it's waiting for a signal you can't find.

And still, life demands that you keep moving. So you do.

You wake up groggy, shake it off, and carry on.
You convince yourself this phase will pass.
You tell yourself this is normal for someone with your workload, your
responsibilities, your life.

After all, everyone gets tired. Everyone has stress.
So why make a problem out of this?

Because the truth is simple: the collapse is already underway.

Not because of one bad night, but because the system inside you, your
nervous system, hormones, rhythms, emotional load, has begun drifting away
from alignment. And sleep, unlike performance or willpower, cannot function
out of alignment for long.

The early stages of sleep loss don't feel like a crisis.
They feel like "not a big deal."

That's why most people miss the signs.
That's why they don't intervene until it's an emergency.

By the time someone finally admits something is wrong, they've often reached
the point where nights feel unpredictable, mornings feel unstable, and their
confidence in their own body starts to slip.

The collapse is silent.
Gradual.
Invisible from the outside.

But once it starts, it rarely reverses on its own.

Sleep is one of the first systems to break when we're overloaded, and the last
one we notice slipping. By the time we realize how fragile it's become,
exhaustion is no longer just physical. It's emotional, cognitive, and deeply
personal.

Because losing sleep doesn't just feel like losing rest.
It feels like losing control.

Section 2: How Stress Accumulates in the Nervous System

Stress doesn't hit all at once either.

Just like sleep, it builds in layers, quietly, gradually, invisibly, until it becomes something you physically feel in your body.

Most people imagine stress as a spike: a rough day, a tense conversation, a deadline, an argument. But the most damaging stress isn't the kind you notice. It's the kind that never fully leaves your system.

Every time your mind shifts into worrying, planning, reacting, or protecting, your nervous system takes note. And when those moments pile up, day after day, month after month, year after year, you stop returning to baseline. You start living in a constant state of "almost alert," even after the immediate threat is gone.

This is how stress accumulates:

- One small pressure. Then another.

- A bit of tension in the shoulders.

- A tightening in breath.

- A faster heartbeat during moments that never bothered you before.

- A mind that runs even when the environment is calm.

Without realizing it, your nervous system begins operating at a higher baseline, one where "relaxed" doesn't feel relaxing anymore, and "tired" doesn't automatically trigger rest. You're trying to sleep in a body that thinks it needs to stay ready.

Stress changes your physiology:

- Your cortisol rises at the wrong times.

- Your heart rate stays too high at night.

- Your mind anticipates problems even in silence.

- Your muscles hold tension long after the day ends.

- Your breath becomes shallow and fast.

- Your internal alarm never fully turns off.

This isn't character.
It isn't weakness.
It isn't a mindset problem.

It's biology.

Your nervous system stores experiences. It remembers pressure, conflict, and emotional strain far longer than your conscious mind does. It processes everything, even the small moments you think you brushed off.

Over time, this accumulation creates a state many people never name:

Hyperarousal.

It's not anxiety.
Not a panic attack.
Not classic "fear."

It's the inability to transition from "on" to "off."

You might not feel stressed, but your body is acting like it needs to stay alert. You go through your day functioning, performing, handling responsibilities, while your nervous system is constantly scanning, preparing, anticipating.

And when night comes, when the world slows down and your responsibilities fade, that internal alertness becomes loud.

That's why stress shows up at night even when you think you're fine during the day.
That's why your mind decides 2 AM is the perfect time to revisit everything you forgot, everything you fear, and everything you haven't resolved.

You're not "bad at relaxing."
You're not "too intense."
You're not "wired wrong."

You're carrying more than your nervous system was designed to handle without recovery.

In that state, sleep isn't just difficult; it becomes biologically blocked.
Your mind and body aren't aligned.
Your systems are working against each other.

Stress that accumulates doesn't dissolve on its own. It embeds itself in your sleep cycle, stretching the time it takes to drift off, shortening the time you stay asleep, and amplifying the impact of even minor disruptions.

Here's the hidden truth most people never learn:

You don't lose sleep just because you're stressed.
You lose sleep because your nervous system never gets the chance to stand down.

Section 3: My Early Signs, Tension, Irritability, Hypervigilance

Looking back, the signs were there long before the sleepless nights, long before I admitted anything was wrong. But like most high performers, I normalized symptoms that should have been warnings.

The first sign was tension.

Not the kind that comes and goes, but a constant, low-level tightness in my shoulders, neck, and chest. I blamed work, training, responsibility, everything except the truth. My body was in a permanent state of readiness, and I didn't recognize it because I had lived that way for so long it felt familiar.

Then came irritability.

Subtle at first, shorter answers, less patience, quicker reactions. Small things bothered me more than they used to. Conversations took more energy. Noise felt louder. Frustration arrived faster. Even when I wasn't angry, I carried an internal pressure that made me feel slightly out of sync with myself.

I wasn't unhappy. I wasn't depressed.
But I wasn't fully myself either.

Then there was hypervigilance, a word I didn't use then but one that perfectly describes what I felt.

It's the sense that your mind is always scanning, always preparing, always running scenarios in the background. Not panic, strategy. Not fear, survival instinct. Not nervousness, awareness sharpened into a blade.

In the beginning, it felt like an advantage.

I was alert. Focused. Ready.
The kind of hyperawareness that builds businesses and protects families.
The kind that comes from growing up in unstable environments where being caught off guard never felt safe.

But the problem with living that way is simple:

Your body doesn't know the difference between vigilance for survival and vigilance for productivity.

It only knows vigilance.

And vigilance is the enemy of sleep.

At the time, I didn't understand that these were early indicators that my sleep system, the emotional, biological, and behavioral parts of it, was drifting out of alignment. I didn't realize that carrying tension during the day meant my body never returned to neutral at night. I didn't see that irritability was a sign of nervous system overload. I didn't know hypervigilance was turning into a 24/7 state of readiness that would eventually make rest feel impossible.

To me, these changes were just part of the grind.

Part of being someone who carried weight others didn't see.
Part of being responsible, ambitious, driven.
Part of living life at a relentless pace.

Like a lot of people, I mistook these symptoms for personality traits:

- Tension meant I was hardworking.

- Irritability meant I was focused.

- Hypervigilance meant I was sharp.

In reality, there were subtle signals that my mind and body were drifting away from recovery mode altogether.

I wish I could say I recognized the signs early and corrected them.
I didn't.

I brushed them off.
I moved faster.
I worked harder.

I told myself the tension would fade, the irritability would ease, the vigilance would quiet once things "slowed down."

They didn't.

Instead, they grew, quietly, consistently, predictably.

Those early signs didn't break me, but they built the foundation for the sleepless nights that followed. They created the environment where sleep became something I had to chase instead of something that came naturally.

And like most people, I didn't realize what was happening until I was already deep in the cycle.

Section 4: The Emotional Cost of Pretending You're Fine

One of the heaviest burdens a person can carry is the need to appear unshakable while quietly falling apart. For many of us, men especially, high performers especially, that burden becomes a way of life.

We become experts at hiding fatigue behind productivity, stress behind discipline, and emotional strain behind a practiced, steady face.

In the early stages of losing sleep, I wasn't worried about my emotional health.
I worried about performance.
About responsibility.
About showing up the way people expected me to.

Because I could still function, I decided that meant I was fine.

But functioning is not the same as being well.

You can be productive and still be unraveling inside.

You can move through your day and still be carrying emotional weight your system can no longer handle.

The emotional cost of sleeplessness starts long before you understand what's happening. It begins the moment you start pretending.

Pretending you're not tired.
Pretending the irritability is just stress.
Pretending the tension is normal.
Pretending the mental fog is just "a long day."
Pretending the nights aren't getting harder.
Pretending the mornings aren't getting heavier.

Pretending is exhausting.
In some ways, more exhausting than the lack of sleep itself.

Because when you pretend, you split it into two versions:

- The version the world sees: focused, committed, reliable, high functioning.

- The version you live privately: drained, overwhelmed, disconnected, running on fumes.

Carrying both is like walking with a quiet fracture. It doesn't stop you from moving, but every step wears you down more than the last.

The emotional cost showed up in places I didn't expect:

- **My patience shortened.**
  Conversations that once felt easy now required effort. Little things irritated me because I had no internal space left to absorb them.

- **My presence faded.**
  I was there physically, but mentally I often felt a few steps removed, like a spectator in my own life.

- **My joy dulled.**
  Good moments, time with family, wins at work, small celebrations, felt muted, like I was experiencing them through foggy glass.

- **My resilience weakened.**
  Things that once rolled off now lingered. Minor setbacks took longer to shake. Small problems felt larger than they were.

- **I stopped confiding in people.**
  Not because I didn't trust them, but because admitting something was wrong, it felt like failure. I didn't have the energy to explain why I felt off.

The tougher you are, the more pressure you feel to maintain the image of toughness. So you hold it in, believing discipline will eventually fix what's slipping.

But discipline doesn't repair an overloaded nervous system.
It doesn't resolve physiological misalignment.
It doesn't quiet a mind locked in a protective loop.

The more you pretend, the more you internalize the belief that you *should* be able to handle this. That belief becomes its own emotional trap:

- If you can't sleep, you blame yourself.

- If your mood dips, you blame yourself.

- If you're not as sharp, you blame yourself.

- If you're exhausted, you blame yourself.

None of this is a moral failing.
It's not a character flaw.
It's not a lack of strength.

It's biology fighting biology.
A nervous system moving out of alignment.
Hormones firing at the wrong time.
Emotional strain your body can't regulate because sleep, the core of emotional regulation, is collapsing underneath you.

When your nights fall apart, your days begin to leak.

The emotional cost of pretending you're fine is that you slowly lose the connection between who you are and how you feel. You become less grounded, less steady, less able to return to calm. Your world narrows. Your capacity shrinks. Your confidence slips in ways you don't talk about.

And yet, on the surface, life continues.

You still work.
You still lead.
You still show up.
You still perform.

But internally…

You're holding everything together with tension instead of stability.

That's the real emotional cost of sleeplessness: it quietly steals pieces of you until the person you're performing as no longer matches the person you feel yourself becoming.

Section 5: How Modern Life Disrupts the Natural Sleep State

Human beings were never designed to live the way we do today.

Our physiology is ancient, built for natural light, predictable rhythms, physical exertion, slower pace, and true downtime. Modern life pulls us in the opposite direction. It turns our days into nonstop current and our nights into an extension of that momentum.

It slowly erodes the conditions that make natural sleep possible.

Most people think they have "insomnia," but what they often have is a lifestyle misaligned with their biology.

We sleep in a world that never shuts off.

We live under artificial light long after sunset.
We stare into screens inches from our faces.
We scroll before bed to "wind down" but end up stimulating our brain into alertness.

We eat later.
Work later.

Respond faster.
Think harder.

We carry our entire social circle and workload in our pockets. We're expected
to be available, reachable, responsive, always.

Our nervous system wasn't built for this level of constant stimulation. And
that overstimulation disrupts every layer of the sleep process.

- **Light** confuses our biological clock.
  Blue light from screens delays melatonin release, shifting the timing
  of sleep. We call ourselves "night owls" as if it's a personality type,
  not a conditioned response.

- **Technology** disrupts internal silence.
  Notifications train our nervous system to stay alert even when we're
  "off." Our minds get used to scanning for input, even in the dark.

- **Stress** doesn't get discharged.
  We move from one task to the next without pause. We treat
  "downtime" as time to scroll. That isn't rest; it's micro-stimulation.

- **Our days lack rhythm.**
  We drink caffeine too late.
  Eat too close to bedtime.
  Exercise erratically.
  Work at unpredictable hours.

Our brains rely on consistency to time sleep hormones, but our schedules are
anything but consistent.

We've also normalized being exhausted.

People brag about running on four hours of sleep.
Being "busy" is a badge of honor.
Exhaustion is framed as proof of ambition.

This culture trains us to dismiss fatigue instead of respecting it, to push
through imbalance instead of correcting it. We confuse mental toughness with
self-neglect.

But sleep doesn't care about hustle, deadlines, or ambition.
It doesn't respond to your intentions.
It responds to alignment.

The biggest misconception of all is that people blame themselves. When sleep becomes difficult, most assume they're "bad sleepers" or "too stressed," or that something is wrong with their willpower. They don't realize their environment, habits, schedule, and tech have been rewiring their sleep systems for years.

The truth is this:

Modern life has separated you from the conditions your body needs to sleep the way it was designed to.

It's not your fault.
It's not a lack of discipline.
It's not a flaw in your character.

It's a mismatch between a nervous system thousands of years old and a modern world only decades old.

Because the disruption happens slowly and invisibly, most people don't understand why sleep becomes such a struggle. They just know:

- They feel tired all the time.

- Their minds won't slow down.

- They wake in the night and don't know why.

- They dread bedtime more than they look forward to it.

They think something is wrong *with them*, when in reality something is wrong with the way their environment interacts with their biology.

This isn't weakness.
It's misalignment.

And misalignment can be corrected, but only once you understand what you're working against.

Section 6: Why People Blame Themselves for Something Physiological

When sleep starts to fall apart, most people don't look outward. They look inward.

They blame their discipline, their stress, their personality, and their willpower. They assume they're doing something wrong, that they're weak, not tough enough, not calm enough, not balanced enough.

Because sleep is such a deeply internal experience, the shame becomes internal too.

But here's the truth:

Most sleep problems aren't psychological failures.
They're physiological ones.

Your body is running a system you don't consciously control:

- Hormone timing

- Circadian alignment

- Heart rate variability

- Oxygen levels

- Core temperature

- Nervous system arousal

- Autonomic activation

- Inflammatory response

When even one of these begins to drift, sleep becomes unstable.
When several go off course at once, sleep can feel nearly impossible.

Because none of this is visible in the moment, you don't see biology breaking down. You just see the surface symptoms: irritability, fatigue, restlessness, tension, poor focus, a mind that won't slow down.

Those feel psychological.
So you decide the problem must be you.

I did the same thing.

For a long time, I believed my sleep issues were purely emotional: tension, hypervigilance, responsibility, the constant fight to hold everything together. And at first, they were. My sleep collapsed from the inside out.

But over time, something deeper started happening, something I didn't understand and didn't want to face.

My body began to break down biologically.

It started quietly:

- Waking up gasping for air and calling it "stress"

- Feeling tired no matter how many hours I spent in bed

- Sudden jerks or micro-awakenings I didn't remember

- A heaviness in my chest at night

- Morning headaches that didn't match how I felt mentally

- Fatigue that felt physical, not emotional

I didn't connect any of it to sleep.
I told myself I was overworked.
That I needed a better routine.
That I had built a life with too much pressure.

I blamed my mindset.
I blamed my stress.
I blamed my habits.

What I never considered, what many people never consider, is this:

Sometimes your sleep disorder isn't primarily psychological.
Sometimes the machine of your body isn't functioning the way it should.

As the months went on, the physical symptoms got harder to ignore.

My breathing at night became irregular.
I woke up feeling like I'd run a marathon.

My energy tanked in ways discipline couldn't fix.
My body felt like it was stuck at half-capacity despite maximum effort.

Eventually, I had to face it:
My biology was now part of the problem.

Getting evaluated led to something I had resisted for years: a CPAP machine.

It was humbling. It was uncomfortable. It was a reminder that even the strongest people can break physically. But it was also the moment I finally saw the full picture:

Sleep is not just mindset.
It's not just discipline.
It's not just stress.

Sleep is a biological system first.
And biology always wins.

That realization reshaped everything I believed about sleep.

It showed me that people aren't to blame for their exhaustion. They're trapped inside systems, behavioral, emotional, biological, that have drifted out of alignment.

Most people suffer silently because they believe the lie that sleep problems mean something is wrong with them as human beings.

But sleep issues don't define character.
They reveal physiology.

You're not weak for struggling to sleep.
You're not broken because you need help.
You're not failing because your body needs support.

And you're not alone.

If anything, the fact that you've made it this far, functioning, pushing, showing up, carrying what you carry, is proof of your strength.

The problem isn't you.
The problem is that nobody taught you how sleep actually works, how the

systems inside you interact, and how to rebuild what's been slowly falling apart.

This book exists to change that.

Now that you understand how the collapse begins, we can start the real journey, not just to *understand* sleep, but to restore it.

Chapter 2: Why Sleep Advice Failes

By the time most people start seriously searching for sleep advice, they're already tired enough to try anything.

They've done the casual Googling.
They've heard the podcasts.
They've read the threads.
They've listened to friends.

"Have you tried magnesium?"
"Cut your caffeine."
"Wear blue-light glasses."
"Meditation changed everything for me."
"Just don't look at your phone after 9PM."

On paper, none of this sounds unreasonable. Some of it is even good advice.

But here's the problem:
for a lot of people, it doesn't work. Or it works for a few days, a week, maybe a month, and then collapses under the weight of real life.

When you're already exhausted, nothing is more demoralizing than doing "all the right things" and still staring at the ceiling at 2 AM.

It's easy, from the outside, to assume people with sleep problems just haven't found the right trick, or aren't trying hard enough, or aren't consistent enough.

The truth is very different.

Most sleep advice fails for one simple reason:

It wasn't built for *you*.
It was built for an imaginary, average nervous system living in an imaginary, average life.

And your reality is not average.

Section 1: The Myth of Universal "Sleep Hacks"

If you've ever struggled to sleep, you know exactly how desperate the nights can become. And desperate people will try anything, which is why the world is flooded with advice, hacks, tips, tricks, rules, and rituals that all promise one thing:

"If you do this, you'll sleep."

For years, I believed that too.

I tried every suggestion that crossed my path. People meant well, friends, doctors, articles, podcasts, all convinced they had found the magic shortcut. And because I was exhausted, I listened. I followed their rules with the discipline I used everywhere else in my life.
But something strange happened:

Every new "hack" only made me feel more broken.

It wasn't that the advice was harmful. It just wasn't designed for *me*. It wasn't designed for everything I had lived through, everything my nervous system carried, everything my biology was fighting against. But back then, I didn't know that. All I knew was that I was trying, and failing.

And failing at sleep feels personal.

I remember one night in particular when I followed a perfectly structured, influencer-approved "bedtime routine." I turned off my phone early. I dimmed the lights. I sat quietly. I drank the herbal tea. I took the warm shower. All the steps, in the right order, at the right time.

My body didn't care.

I laid there, eyes open, frustration rising like heat from the mattress. Every minute that passed felt like a punch to the gut. The routine wasn't the problem. The expectation was. I believed that if I checked every box, sleep would reward me. But sleep doesn't bargain. It doesn't respond to rituals performed out of fear. It doesn't respond to hacks that ignore the reasons your system is misaligned in the first place.

Here's the truth I didn't understand at the time:

Most sleep advice works, just not for the person who truly needs it.

Sleep hacks are built for people whose systems are mostly aligned, people who simply need a nudge, not a rescue. They're written for people who already sleep decently but want to sleep *better*. They're not built for the person staring at the ceiling at 3 AM with a nervous system stuck in overdrive. They're not built for people with trauma history, high-pressure careers, nighttime hypervigilance, biological misalignment, or years of accumulated stress.

They certainly weren't built for me.

But I didn't know that then. Instead, I blamed myself.

When a hack didn't work, I assumed I did it wrong. When a routine failed, I tightened the routine. When a technique flopped, I performed it with even more precision.
Every failure chipped away at my confidence, until I wasn't just exhausted, I felt defeated.

The myth of universal sleep hacks convinces people that sleep is a simple equation:

Do this = get that.

But sleep doesn't respond to formulas. It responds to systems, emotional, biological, behavioral, and if even one of those systems is off, all the hacks in the world won't reach the root.
When the advice failed, I thought *I* was the failure.

But I wasn't the problem.
The advice was too shallow for the depth of what I was living.

And as you'll see, this is where most people get stuck, trapped in a cycle of trying harder, blaming themselves, and sinking deeper into frustration.

Because sleep is not one thing.
And any solution that treats it like one was never going to work.

Section 2: Why "Just Relax" Is Psychologically Impossible for Wired Minds

If you've struggled with sleep, you already know the phrase that shows up sooner or later, usually said with a gentle shrug:

"Just relax."

People mean well when they say it. They think they're offering comfort or a reminder to take pressure off. But if you've ever been lying in bed with your heart pounding, your thoughts looping, your chest tight, your mind buzzing as if someone flipped every switch inside you to *high*, you know exactly how hollow that advice sounds.

Relaxation isn't a command.
It's a state.
And a wired nervous system doesn't enter that state because someone tells it to.

When your system has been running hot for years, *"just relax"* doesn't feel supportive. It feels like a judgment. Like someone is pointing out something you should be able to do but can't. It makes you feel defective in a way you don't say out loud.

I remember nights when I genuinely tried to follow that advice.
I'd close my eyes, take a slow breath, and think:

Alright, calm down. Let go. Fix this.

Within seconds I'd feel the opposite happening.
My breathing would tighten.
My thoughts would pick up speed.
My chest would tense like I was bracing for impact.
I'd start evaluating every sensation, studying myself, trying to catch proof that I was becoming calmer.

Nothing makes your body more tense than trying to prove you're not tense.

And when it didn't work, the internal dialogue got harsher:

Why can't I relax?
What's wrong with me?

Why is my body acting like this?
Why can't I do something so simple?

This is the part nobody talks about:
"Just relax" doesn't just fail, it makes you feel like the failure.

But the truth is simple:

Relaxation isn't a mental choice.
It's a physiological shift.

Relaxation happens when your nervous system receives enough signals of safety to release its grip. When your internal alarms stop firing. When your body stops scanning for threats. When your mind stops anticipating what could go wrong.

But when you've spent years, or decades, in high-alert mode, your body doesn't respond to gentleness. It responds to *evidence.*

Your system needs proof:

- that the environment is safe
- that your breath has slowed
- that your heart rate has softened
- that your day has truly ended
- that you are no longer required to perform, fix, protect, or anticipate

Without that evidence, your body does exactly what it was built to do: **stay alert.**
Not because you're weak.
Not because you're "bad at relaxing."
Not because something is wrong with your mind.

Your body is doing its job.

It's protecting you from a threat that no longer exists, but that your nervous system still remembers.

And if you've lived a life where you've had to be strong, tough, prepared, resilient, or hyper-responsible, you know exactly how easily that protective state becomes permanent.

My nights were shaped by that permanence.
Even when the world outside was calm, the world inside me stayed ready.
I wasn't anxious, I was conditioned.

And this is what most people never learn:

You cannot think your way out of a physiological state.

You can want rest.
You can long for it.
You can desperately beg your mind and body to give you one peaceful night.

But wanting rest and being able to *enter* rest are two different things.

When someone tells you to relax without understanding the biology underneath, they are offering a solution that works only for people whose systems are already aligned. People who are tired, not wired. People who can flip into calm because their body still remembers how.

For the rest of us, "just relax" is like standing at the bottom of a mountain you've climbed your whole life and being told to simply float.

Your system needs retraining, not reminders.
Safety signals, not slogans.
Alignment, not pressure.
A method, not a mantra.

Nothing is wrong with you.
The problem is that the world keeps handing people psychological instructions for a physiological state.

Sleep doesn't begin with "relax."
Sleep begins when your body believes it no longer has to protect you.

Section 3: Advice Overload and the Paradox of Trying Harder

At some point in your struggle with sleep, you probably did what I did: you started searching for answers. It always begins innocently, one bad night, then two, then a week that feels off. You look for simple tips. You scroll through articles. You listen to podcasts. You try the tricks your friends swear by.

What starts as curiosity quickly becomes a full-time job.

By the time most people realize something is actually wrong, they're buried under a mountain of advice. Every expert, influencer, and wellness blogger has a different opinion. Everyone claims their solution is the "real" fix.

And you, exhausted and desperate, try to follow all of it.

At first, the advice feels empowering. Busy people love clear directions. We love strategies and structure, the idea that if we can just execute well enough, the problem will disappear.

But sleep doesn't respond to effort that way.

The harder you push, the worse it gets.

This is the hidden trap nobody warns you about:
the moment you turn sleep into a task, you turn your nervous system into a supervisor. And suddenly, you're not falling asleep, you're performing at falling asleep.

That shift changes everything.

When Sleep Becomes a Job Instead of a Process

You know you're in the trap when nighttime begins to feel like a project. You start adding rules to your evenings:

- No screens after 9:00

- No food after 7:00

- Drink this tea

- Turn on this sound

- Take that supplement

- Stretch, meditate, journal

- Don't think about tomorrow

- Don't think about not thinking

- Don't focus on trying

- Don't focus on not trying

You go to bed with instructions instead of instincts.

And the moment you start managing your way through sleep, something inside you tightens. You start monitoring yourself, checking whether you're "doing it right," watching for signs that your body is responding.

You lie there waiting for sleep to happen, as if sleep were something you could summon by following the perfect formula.

But that's not how sleep works.

Sleep is a surrender, not a strategy.

The paradox is this:
the more effort you invest in sleeping, the more alert your system becomes.

Trying harder *activates* the very part of your brain that needs to deactivate.

My Own Descent Into the Advice Spiral

I went through the same cycle. The more nights I struggled, the more I chased solutions. I followed every checklist I could find, hoping one would finally fix the problem. But instead of getting better, I became more aware of every sensation in my body.

I noticed my breathing.
My heart rate.
The way my chest felt before bed.
The exact moment a thought would loop.
The temperature of the room.
The way the blankets felt.
How long it took before I felt "sleepy enough."

It became an obsession, disguised as self-discipline.

But underneath the rituals, routines, and rules, my nervous system wasn't softening. It was becoming more vigilant. Every piece of advice I collected, every "hack," every sleep product, every lifestyle tweak, added more pressure to the process.

Nighttime became a test I couldn't pass.

And every failed attempt made me feel more defective.
More confused.
More convinced that something inside me was broken.

But the truth was simpler:

The advice wasn't wrong.
It just wasn't right for the state I was in.

When you're deeply wired, stressed, or misaligned, advice that's meant for mild sleep trouble becomes fuel for a bigger fire.

Why Advice Overload Makes Things Worse

Most sleep tips assume your nervous system is calm enough to respond.

But if you're already overwhelmed, stressed, or stuck in hyperarousal, the advice turns into pressure:

- "I have to do this right."

- "If this doesn't work, I'm in trouble."

- "What am I missing?"

- "Why am I failing at something so basic?"

- "What happens if I don't sleep tonight?"

Those thoughts fire up your stress circuits.

Suddenly, the help becomes another demand.
Another task.
Another invisible weight.

Trying harder activates the system that's supposed to turn off.

That's why people can meditate for twenty minutes, drink sleepy tea, take magnesium, use perfect lighting, and still lie awake thinking:

"Why isn't this working?"

It's because all of that "advice" is happening on the outside, while the real problem is happening on the inside.

The Real Issue Is Not Lack of Advice, It's Lack of Alignment

Most people don't have an information problem.
They have an alignment problem.

Their behavioral system, biological system, and emotional system are not working together. They're pulling in different directions. And no amount of tips can sync up systems that haven't been understood first.

This is why sleep advice fails.
Not because it's bad advice, but because it isn't personalized to the state of the person using it.

That's what the Dreameaz Method was built to change, by helping people stop chasing tactics and start restoring alignment.

You'll see as you move deeper into the book:

Sleep doesn't return when you do more.
Sleep returns when you stop fighting your body and start understanding it.

And that begins by letting go of the pressure to "perform" your way into rest.

Section 4: Why Medication Helps Some but Fails Many

For most people, medication is the point they reach when the nights stop making sense. It isn't the first step. It's the step you take when you've already tried everything else, the routines, the hacks, the breathwork, the teas, the podcasts, the supplements, and nothing changes.

I reached that step too.

At first, I started small, the same way most people do.
Something over the counter. Something harmless. Something that promised
to "nudge" my sleep in the right direction. And for a brief moment, I believed
it worked. I fell asleep faster, and that felt like hope.

But mornings told the truth.

I woke up groggy, foggy, and somehow more exhausted than the night
before. It took longer to shake off the heaviness. My mind felt thick. My body
felt slow. But I convinced myself it was better than lying awake.

When that stopped working, I tried something stronger. Then something
stronger than that. And eventually I found myself holding prescriptions I
swore I'd never need. Each one promised rest. Each one delivered something
that *looked* like sleep on paper, hours unaccounted for, consciousness shut off,
but inside, something felt wrong.

I would wake with the same tension in my chest.
The same racing mind.
The same fatigue that sat deep in my bones.

It took me a long time to understand why.

Medication can make you unconscious,
but unconsciousness is not sleep.

Real sleep is an active process, a biological dance the brain orchestrates
through stages of repair, regulation, emotional processing, memory sorting,
hormonal balancing, and nervous system recalibration.
Medication doesn't guide your brain through that process. It simply forces the
lights off.

And at first, forced darkness feels like relief.
But over time, it becomes something else:
a substitute your body never asked for.

I started waking feeling as if I'd missed something essential.
Like my brain had been shut down instead of restored.
Like the night had passed, but I hadn't traveled through it.

That's the part most people never realize:

Medication doesn't fail because people are weak.
It fails because it can't do the job natural sleep is designed to do.

This doesn't mean medication is bad.
There are moments in life, acute stress, trauma, true crisis, when it becomes the safety net that keeps you functioning. Sometimes it's necessary. Sometimes it saves you.

But medication is a bridge, not a solution.

It can quiet the symptoms for a night.
It cannot realign the systems that broke in the first place.

It cannot:

- lower nighttime cortisol

- repair your circadian rhythm

- retrain a wired nervous system

- heal emotional patterns

- correct breathing disruptions

- restore natural deep sleep

It cannot teach your body how to sleep,
it can only distract it from the fact that it can't.

Looking back, I realized my body wasn't asking for sedation. It was asking for alignment. It was begging for the chance to reset, to settle, to breathe, to recover in the way human bodies were built to recover.

No pill can give you that.
Only a recalibrated system can.

Medication didn't fail me.
It simply couldn't do the job I needed it to do.
And it can't do that job for millions of people who rely on it out of desperation.

Not because they're broken,
but because medication was never designed to fix misalignment.

It only covers it.

And if you've felt that same sinking realization, that the pills are getting stronger, but the mornings are getting worse, you're not alone.

Your body isn't rejecting help.
It's asking for the *right* kind of help.

And that's where this method begins.

Section 5: The Missing Link: True Personalization

There comes a moment in every sleep struggle when you start wondering if you're the only person whose body refuses to follow the rules. You've tried the routines. You've tried the advice. You've tried the supplements. You've tried the medication. You've followed every checklist, every protocol, every "10 steps to better sleep" article written by someone who probably slept eight hours the night before.

And still, your nights fall apart.

That's the moment most people decide something must be wrong with *them*. I know that feeling well, the sinking sense that your body is the exception, that your mind is the outlier, that you're somehow built differently from everyone who can close their eyes and drift off like it's nothing.

But the truth is far simpler, and far less personal:

Sleep advice doesn't fail because you're broken.
It fails because you're unique.

Every piece of generic advice assumes the same thing, that all sleep problems come from the same root, and therefore the same fix should work for everyone. But sleep doesn't work that way. Sleep is not a one-system process. It's three systems working in harmony:

- **Behavioral** (the habits, schedules, rhythms)

- **Biological** (the hormones, temperature, breathing, circadian timing)

- **Emotional** (the nervous system, stress load, trauma patterns)

And no two people have the same combination of misalignment across those systems.

Some people struggle because their **behavioral system** is chaotic, too much light, too many screens, caffeine too late, no routine.
Others struggle because their **biological system** is misfiring, cortisol spikes at night, melatonin suppressed, circadian rhythm drifting, oxygen dropping.
Others struggle because their **emotional system** is overloaded, hypervigilance, unresolved stress, anxiety loops, trauma triggers.
And many people, like me, struggle because **all three** slowly drift out of sync over years.

How could a single hack fix all of that?

How could one piece of advice address systems that require completely different solutions?

It can't.
And that's why people fail.
Not because of the advice,
but because of the mismatch between the advice
and their actual internal system.

For years, I didn't know any of this. I approached sleep the same way I approached business, training, leadership, with effort, discipline, and force. I believed that if I worked hard enough at relaxing, at controlling my mind, at following the rules, I'd eventually "win" at sleep.

But sleep doesn't reward effort.
It rewards alignment.

And alignment looks different for every person.

For some, it means fixing the timing of their biology.
For others, it means repairing a nervous system stuck in survival mode.
For others, it means reshaping the behaviors that unknowingly trigger wakefulness.

Most people need a combination, priorities, adjustments, and recalibrations
across the three systems.

That's the missing link,
and the reason generic advice fails so many people.

You don't need a better routine.
You don't need stronger discipline.
You don't need more supplements or a more rigid schedule.
You don't need to try harder.

You need to know *which system is breaking your sleep*
and how to realign *that* system without fear, force, or guesswork.

The Dreameaz Method exists for this exact reason,
not to give you more advice,
but to help you understand *you.*

What your body needs.
What your mind needs.
What your biology needs.
What your unique history has shaped.
What your system is trying to tell you.

Because once you see your sleep through the lens of your own systems,
not through someone else's checklist,
everything finally starts to make sense.

This is where frustration becomes clarity.
Where shame dissolves.
Where exhaustion feels solvable.
Where the body begins to trust itself again.

And for the first time in a long time,
sleep stops feeling like a fight
and starts feeling like something that belongs to you again.

Chapter 3: Sleep Is Not One Thing

Section 1: Introduction to The Dreameaz Three-System Model™

For most of my life, I believed sleep worked like a light switch.
You flipped it on at the end of the day, and your mind obeyed.
If it didn't, you pushed harder, more discipline, more control, more effort.

That mindset worked for almost everything else in my life.
It never worked for sleep.

For years, I kept asking myself the wrong question:
"What is wrong with me?"

It wasn't until much later, after nights that felt endless, after mornings that felt heavier than they should, after trying routines, supplements, advice, and discipline, that I realized something I had never even considered:

Sleep isn't one thing.

It's a constellation of processes, patterns, and physiological rhythms that depend on each other.
And when even one-part drifts, the entire structure becomes unstable.

Looking back, it seems obvious, but at the time it hit me like a revelation:

Sleep doesn't collapse because you're weak.
Sleep collapses because your systems are out of alignment.

The Dreameaz Three-System Model™ was born from that realization, not from theory, not from textbooks, but from the lived experience of having those systems fall apart, one by one, until I finally saw what was happening beneath the surface.

What Finally Changed Everything

I remember the exact moment I knew I was missing something fundamental.

It was late.
The house was quiet.
Everyone else was asleep.

I had done everything "right" that day:

No caffeine.
No screens.
Workout finished early.
Evening routine checked off like a checklist.
Breathing exercises, stretching, reading, a perfect script.

Yet the moment I laid down, my body felt like it was preparing for impact.
My chest tight.
My mind was wide awake.
A pressure behind my eyes that felt more like readiness than fatigue.

Nothing made sense.

I wasn't emotionally spiraling.
I wasn't overthinking.
I wasn't having a stressful day.

Still, my body refused to shift into rest.

I sat up, frustrated and confused, and whispered something I didn't mean to say aloud:

"Which part of me isn't cooperating?"

That single question was the reason everything eventually changed.

Because the truth is, there wasn't one part.
There were *three*.
Three systems that had been drifting out of alignment for years, so quietly, so gradually, that I didn't recognize what was happening until the collapse was complete.

Sleep Depends on Three Interlocking Systems

Most people think sleep is controlled by mindset or routine or the amount of stress they're carrying. But the real picture is much more complex, and much more hopeful.

Sleep emerges when **three systems** align:

- **The Behavioral System**, everything you do

- **The Biological System**, everything your body does

- **The Emotional System**, everything your nervous system interprets

These systems operate like gears inside a machine.
When they move together, sleep is seamless.
When they drift apart, sleep becomes fragmented, shallow, unpredictable, or impossible.

What makes sleep so fragile is that these gears don't break loudly.
They slip quietly.

You don't notice the first degree of misalignment.
You barely notice the second.
By the third, you're fighting your own physiology in the middle of the night, wondering why nothing works and why you feel like you're losing control.

Why This Model Matters

Most sleep advice focuses on one dimension:

- "Fix your habits."

- "Lower your stress."

- "Support your circadian rhythm."

- "Just disconnect and relax."

None of these are wrong.
They're just incomplete.

You can have perfect habits but be emotionally overloaded.
You can be emotionally stable but biologically disrupted.
You can have a strong biology but chaotic routines.

If one system is misaligned, the others eventually follow.

This is why sleep doesn't fall apart suddenly, it deteriorates.

And it's also why sleep doesn't come back suddenly, it needs realignment.

The Dreameaz Three-System Model™ gives language to what people experience but can't explain:

- Why nighttime feels different than daytime

- Why your mind wakes up when your body wants to rest

- Why routines that used to work suddenly don't

- Why you can feel exhausted but stay wired

- Why some nights feel random though nothing changed

- Why you can function all day but fall apart the moment the lights go out

In my own journey, the model didn't just help me understand sleep.
It helped me understand myself.

Because sleep isn't just about closing your eyes,
it's about everything that happens inside you before you do.

When All Three Systems Drift

Before my sleep collapsed, I thought I was simply tired.
Working too hard.
Living fast.
Taking on more than most.

What I didn't know was that all three systems were slowly separating:

- My **behaviors** were chaotic, late nights, screens, adrenaline-filled days.

- My **biology** was out of rhythm, cortisol spikes, airway collapse, exhaustion deep in my bones.

- My **emotional system** was overloaded, hypervigilance disguised as drive, old trauma patterns, responsibility pressing on my nervous system like weight I didn't know I was carrying.

None of them broke overnight.
They drifted.
Then they drifted further.
And as they pulled away from each other, sleep stopped being something natural, and became something I had to chase.

That's the part most people don't understand:

You don't lose sleep.
You lose alignment.

This Chapter Marks the Turning Point

From here forward, the book changes.
Because now we're not just talking about sleep collapsing,
we're talking about how it can be rebuilt.

In the next sections, I'll break down each system, behavioral, biological, and emotional, with the depth people deserve but almost no one ever receives.

But before we do, I want you to understand one thing clearly:

You are not broken.
Your systems are misaligned.
And misalignment can be corrected.

The moment you understand this model is the moment sleep stops being a mystery
and starts becoming something you can reclaim.

Section 2: The Behavioral System

If you were to step back and watch your own life from a distance, you'd see something you probably never noticed while living it:
your days have been training your nights for years.

Not consciously.
Not intentionally.
But quietly, through small, repeated behaviors that seem harmless on the surface and catastrophic only in hindsight.

The Behavioral System is the first sleep system most people disrupt, long before biology starts misfiring and long before emotions begin tightening their grip. It's the system shaped by the rhythm of your days, the timing of your nights, the habits you repeat without thinking, and the patterns your nervous system absorbs almost by accident.

When this system drifts, it doesn't make a sound.
You don't feel it breaking.
You don't see it shifting.

But one day you wake up and realize it's been pulling your sleep out of alignment for years.

The Life That Trains Your Nights

For most of your life, your days probably looked something like this:

You woke up and immediately stepped into motion.
You solved problems before your feet hit the ground.
You carried responsibility from morning until night.
You pushed through fatigue because slowing down felt dangerous or unearned.
You worked long after your energy told you to stop.
You squeezed tasks into gaps that once belonged to quiet.
You used evenings not as recovery but as catch-up.

Not because you chose this dynamic deliberately,
but because the world you lived in made it feel normal.

This is how most of us drift without realizing it:

We don't notice the moment bedtime becomes the final task of the day instead of the natural end to it.
We don't see that our phones become extensions of our attention.
We don't realize that caffeine becomes a substitute for rest rather than a tool.

We don't understand that bright screens at night slowly rewrite our internal clock.

Every small behavior nudges the nervous system in one direction: **further from rest, deeper into alertness.**

How the Drifting Begins

Behavior shifts in micro-moments:

You start keeping the lights on later.
You answer an email at 10PM because "it'll take 30 seconds."
You scroll for twenty minutes, which becomes forty, which becomes an hour.
You stay up later to catch up on the part of your day you lost to everyone else's needs.
You eat dinner later.
You caffeinate later.
You decompress by stimulating your mind instead of settling it.

You tell yourself none of this is a big deal.
But your nervous system is keeping score.

Your brain is Pavlovian, it learns from repetition.
If the evenings become a second shift, the brain prepares for one.
If nighttime becomes a time for input, the brain gets good at staying alert.
If you habitually wind down by revving the mind, the mind learns that nighttime is performance time, not recovery time.

Little by little, the behaviors of your days teach your nights to stay awake.

The Three Behaviors That Most Quietly Erode Sleep

There are dozens of behavioral disruptors, but three categories do the most damage without people realizing it:

1. Light and Rhythm

You weren't built for screens glowing inches from your face at 11PM.

Yet the modern person exposes their brain to more artificial light at night than any generation before them.

Light delays melatonin.
Light tells the brain the day isn't over.
Light shifts the sleep–wake cycle by hours.

Most people don't recognize this shift because it feels gradual.
But over time, your brain begins treating 10PM like 7PM, and midnight like 9PM.

You're not a "night owl."
You've been conditioned by your environment.

2. Stimulation and Momentum

Everything you consume, work, messages, news, content, adds cognitive velocity.

Your brain ends the day moving as fast as it spent the day learning to move.

If you scroll or multitask or solve problems until the moment you get into bed, your nervous system remains locked in that same gear.
Your body may lie down, but your mind is still sprinting.

People think they have trouble falling asleep.

Most of them have trouble stopping.

3. Inconsistent Timing

Your biology thrives on rhythm, not variety.

But modern life is built on inconsistency:

Irregular wake times.
Irregular meals.
Irregular exercise.
Irregular work blocks.
Irregular downtime.

Your sleep system doesn't know what to expect because it receives different signals every day.

A confused system doesn't shut down predictably.

The Behavioral System Was the First Part of Your Own Sleep to Unravel

When I look back on how my own sleep began to fall apart, this was where the unraveling started, not with trauma, not with stress, not with biology, but with life creeping into the hours that once belonged to rest.

My nights became extensions of my days.
My phone became my last interaction before sleep.
My mind stayed busy because I spent too many hours in states of acceleration.
I "wound down" by absorbing new input instead of releasing old weight.
I treated bedtime like a switch I could flip, ignoring that switches don't exist in human physiology.

The Behavioral System is the first line of defense for sleep.
But when it erodes, everything downstream begins to collapse:

Your biology compensates.
Your emotions compensate.
Your nervous system compensates.

Eventually those systems burn out because they were never meant to carry the load.

Why This System Matters More Than People Realize

The Behavioral System is the only one of the three you can access directly.

You can't consciously change your cortisol curve.
You can't manually trigger melatonin release.
You can't tell your amygdala to relax.

But you *can* change:

When you expose yourself to light
How you transition into evenings
When you eat
When you move
How you decompress

How you end your day
How you signal "We're done for the night"

Your behaviors are the inputs your biology reads.

And if those inputs drift out of alignment, the rest of the system follows.

This is why people blame themselves.
This is why they think they're "bad sleepers."
This is why they feel broken.

But they're not broken.

Their lives are simply teaching their bodies the wrong rhythm.

Section 3: The Biological System

There's a point in every sleep struggle where the body starts speaking louder than the mind, but most people miss it because they've been trained to look inward for the problem, not inward to their biology, but inward to their discipline, their mindset, their stress tolerance. I did the same thing. I blamed my thoughts, my workload, my responsibilities, my drive. I assumed the exhaustion I was feeling was an emotional problem, a cognitive overload, a stress response.

What I didn't understand then, what most people don't understand, is that long before sleep fully collapses, the **body begins shifting in ways you can't see or control**. Biological misalignment doesn't announce itself. It whispers. And like all whispers, it's easy to ignore if you're someone who has spent a lifetime pushing through discomfort.

For years, I didn't consider that biology could be the missing piece. I thought sleep was something you "did," not something your body orchestrated with the precision of a symphony. But biology was working behind the scenes the whole time. And my biology, quietly, steadily, predictably, was beginning to fail.

The Body Has Its Own Clock, And Mine Was Drifting

Your circadian rhythm is ancient. It's older than your personality, older than your habits, older than everything you believe makes you who you are. It sets the timing of sleep, hormones, digestion, body temperature, alertness, recovery, everything.

When it works, you don't notice it.
When it drifts, you feel it in ways that make no sense.

In my case, the shift was microscopic at first:

- I started feeling awake later at night, even when tired.

- I woke up earlier, long before my alarm.

- My energy peaks came at the wrong times.

- My evenings felt wired instead of winding down.

I didn't connect any of this to circadian misalignment. I just told myself, *"It's stress. It'll pass."* But biology doesn't "pass" without intervention. It reorganizes. It compensates. It adapts. And eventually, it breaks.

Cortisol and Melatonin: The Invisible Battle

There's a dance inside the body, cortisol rising in the morning, melatonin rising at night. When that dance goes off rhythm, sleep becomes unpredictable. You feel tired but wired. You feel awake at the wrong times. You lie there wondering why your body is acting like it's preparing for something instead of letting go.

I lived in that pattern for months.

I'd climb into bed wanting nothing more than rest, but the moment the lights went out, something in my body switched on. My mind was active, yes, but beneath that was a deeper, heavier hum, as if my whole system was on the wrong timeline. Cortisol spiking at night. Melatonin delayed. Sleep pressure building but never landing.

You can force discipline.
You can't force hormones.

But I tried anyway, routines, rules, relaxation techniques, all in a body that had quietly flipped its internal clock without my permission.

Temperature: The Silent Gatekeeper of Sleep

People rarely think about temperature when they think about sleep, but your body has to drop in core temperature to transition into the first stages. When it doesn't, your mind doesn't follow.

For me, this showed up as restlessness. Tossing. Turning. Feeling "activated" even when exhausted. Nights where I couldn't find stillness because my body wouldn't release heat the way it should.

I didn't know that chronic stress and constant activation can interfere with the body's ability to cool down at night. I just assumed I was uncomfortable, not misaligned. But every degree matters. When temperature fails to drop, the doorway into sleep narrows to a sliver.

Digestion, Metabolism, and the Cost of Always Being "On"

The modern world pushes our metabolic system far past its design. Eating late, eating fast, eating under stress, the digestive system becomes overloaded. And when digestion is active at night, sleep becomes shallow or fragmented.

This happened to me without me realizing it:

- Late dinners after long workdays.

- Food taken in on the move.

- Meals eaten at the tail end of adrenaline cycles.

These seem harmless in isolation, but biology doesn't treat them as isolated events. Every choice during the day becomes part of the sleep equation at night.

I'd wake up with heaviness in my chest, sluggish mornings, unexplained fatigue, all rooted in a body still digesting when it should have been repairing.

Sleep is not a switch.
It's chemistry.

And chemistry demands order.

Breathing: The Part I Ignored the Longest

There's a kind of fatigue that discipline cannot overcome, the fatigue that comes from a body starved of oxygen for hours every night. I didn't want to believe that was happening to me. I had spent my whole life being strong, being capable, being the one who pushed past limits.

But biology doesn't care who you think you are.

It wasn't until the nights became unbearable, the gasping awake, the choking sensations, the morning headaches, the bone-deep exhaustion that sleep couldn't fix, that I finally understood something was happening inside my body that mindset, toughness, or grit would never resolve.

Sleep-disordered breathing didn't just take my sleep from me. It took pieces of my health, my patience, my clarity. And it happened so gradually that I almost didn't see it until it was crippling.

The CPAP was humbling.
A machine forcing air to keep me alive at night.
A reminder that strength doesn't protect you from physiology.

But in a strange way, that moment restored my power, because it gave me the truth.

The Body Will Always Tell the Truth Before the Mind Will Admit It

Before people struggle to fall asleep, before they wake through the night, before sleep anxiety takes root, the biological system almost always begins to drift:

- Hormones misalign.

- Temperature regulation falters.

- Breathing destabilizes.

- Circadian timing shifts.

- Metabolic strain increases.

- Stress chemicals rise at the wrong times.

The body breaks quietly, long before the mind realizes the collapse is coming.

Looking back, all the signs were there, not emotional signs, not behavioral ones, but biological ones. I didn't lose sleep because something was "wrong with me." I lost sleep because the systems inside me were no longer synchronized.

The Dreameaz approach was born from this revelation:

You cannot fix sleep unless you fix the systems that create it.

And biology, the part of sleep people often ignore, is the system that almost always begins the collapse.

You don't need to fight your mind.
You need to work with your physiology.

Because when the body remembers how to sleep, the mind follows.

Section 4: The Emotional System

For most of my life, I thought sleep was something the body did on its own, a mechanical function, like a machine powering down. I didn't understand that sleep depends on what the mind is doing long before the lights go out. I didn't realize that your emotional state is one of the strongest forces shaping what happens after your head hits the pillow.

The Emotional System is the most invisible of the three sleep systems, and the easiest to misunderstand. You can see your behaviors. You can measure your biology. But your emotional patterns? Those live behind the face you show the world. They're subtle, layered, and often disguised as "normal personality traits" you've carried for years.

Most people don't realize the emotional system is breaking down until sleep is already slipping away.

And that's exactly why it's so powerful.

The Emotional System: The Quiet Engine Behind Your Nights

The Emotional System governs the mental and feeling-based states that must shift for sleep to occur.

This system includes:

- cognitive load

- rumination patterns

- anticipatory thoughts

- unresolved stress

- emotional triggers

- the stories you tell yourself about sleep

- the pressure you carry from the day into the night

Sleep depends on the body being able to surrender, something many people haven't felt in years.

If your Emotional System is in overdrive, the mind doesn't transition from thinking to drifting. Instead, it clings to control. It replays conversations. It anticipates tomorrow. It reopens old stress you didn't have time to process during the day.

Night becomes a doorway with no door. There's no separation, no release, no shift into quiet.

How the Mind Learns to Stay "On"

Most emotional sleep disruptions don't come from dramatic life events. They come from small, daily patterns the mind begins to rely on without you noticing.

It looks like:

- replaying the day on a loop

- mentally rehearsing tomorrow's responsibilities

- trying to "solve" problems that aren't immediate

- tightening around uncertainty

- keeping score of what went wrong or what might

- revisiting conversations you can't change

The mind thinks it's helping. It doesn't realize it's interfering with the very thing that would help it more than anything else: deep, restorative sleep.

In my own life, this pattern didn't announce itself with panic or fear. It came as thoughtfulness, planning, and responsibility, all things I believed were strengths. But strengths overused become strain. And strain creates emotional momentum that doesn't simply turn off at night.

It's not that you're "overthinking."
It's that your emotional system doesn't trust the off-switch anymore.

The Stories We Tell Ourselves at Night

Every person has an internal narrative that grows louder when the world gets quiet.

Some people worry.
Some rehearse.
Some catastrophize.
Some problem-solve.
Some brace for the next day.
Some wonder if they will sleep at all.

For many, the emotional system becomes conditioned to anticipate failure:

"What if I can't sleep tonight?"
"What if this gets worse?"
"What if tomorrow is ruined?"

These aren't just thoughts. They are emotional imprints, tiny signals to the brain that something is uncertain, unsafe, or unresolved. And when the brain senses uncertainty, it responds with vigilance.

This is why so many people say they can be exhausted all day but suddenly feel alert at night. The mind isn't energized. It's guarding.

In my own nights, it started subtly. The moment the lights dimmed, my mind became the loudest thing in the room. Not emotional turmoil, just activity. Scanning. Planning. Holding tension. Trying to stay one step ahead of a world that asked for a lot.

Nothing felt wrong.
But nothing felt quiet, either.

That's how the emotional system slips out of alignment, not with chaos, but with momentum.

Emotional Carryover: The Weight You Don't Notice Until Bedtime

The emotional system carries the residue of the day. Stress doesn't disappear just because the clock hits 10 PM. The emotional load you didn't process leaks into the moments when your mind becomes still enough to notice it.

This is why:

- you can feel fine during the day and overwhelmed at night

- your thoughts speed up the moment you lie down

- small worries grow larger in the dark

- emotions you ignored show up uninvited

- old stress resurfaces without warning

The emotional system doesn't operate on your schedule. It operates when the environment finally stops demanding your attention.

That's when it brings everything forward.

Why the Emotional System Is the Final Barrier to Sleep

Of all three systems, the Emotional System is the one most people try to override through sheer willpower.

They tell themselves:
"Stop thinking."

"Calm down."
"Don't worry about it."
"Let it go."

But you can't "command" an emotional state.
You can only create the conditions for it.

When your Emotional System is activated:

- the mind orbits the same thoughts

- the body prepares for action instead of rest

- cortisol rises

- heart rate stays elevated

- breathing becomes shallow

- sleep becomes blocked, not delayed

This is why trying harder to sleep often backfires. Effort activates the emotional system even more.

I've experienced this myself, lying in bed, willing sleep to come, feeling the tension rise as the minutes passed. The harder I tried, the more awake I felt. Not from fear. Not from panic. Just from effort.

Effort and emotion, together, build a wall between you and sleep.

When All Three Systems Interact

The Emotional System never breaks alone. It always affects the other two.

- When emotions run high, the Biological System shifts into alertness.

- When the biology is activated, the Behavioral System compensates with more screens, late nights, or irregular routines.

- When behaviors drift, emotions intensify, frustration, worry, self-blame.

- And the cycle continues, quietly but relentlessly.

In my own case, I didn't realize how these systems were interacting until everything began to show up at once. The emotional load. The biological imbalance. The behaviors that filled the gaps.

It didn't feel catastrophic.
It felt manageable, right until it wasn't.

That's the danger of the emotional system:
You don't feel it failing.
You feel it holding on.

And that illusion delays the very help your nights need most.

Why Understanding the Emotional System Matters

You can fix your behaviors.
You can correct your biology.
You can improve your routines.

But until the Emotional System learns to stand down, no sleep strategy will work consistently.

The emotional system is the final gatekeeper, the part of you that must feel safe, unburdened, and permitted to let go. It decides whether the mind drifts or clings, whether the night becomes healing or another battlefield.

Rebuilding this system isn't about eliminating emotion. It's about creating an internal environment where your emotional world no longer conflicts with your need to sleep.

It's about teaching your system that it's allowed to rest.

And once it learns that,
once the emotional system begins to trust the night again,
the entire architecture of sleep starts to rebuild from the inside out.

Chapter 4: The Behavioral System

Section 1: Light Exposure, Daily Rhythms, and Screens

If you really want to understand why sleep slips away from so many people, you have to start with the simplest truth of all: the human body was built to follow the sun. Every cell, every hormone, every internal rhythm still runs on a pattern older than civilization itself. In the natural world, light means action. Darkness means release. Our biology has always depended on that contrast.

But the world we live in now doesn't honor that contrast at all. We live in a world where the sun never really sets, not for our eyes, not for our brains, and certainly not for our behavior.

For most of my life, I didn't think about light as anything more than a background detail. You flip a switch, you see, you work, you live. But the deeper I fell into my own sleep struggles, the more I realized the truth I'd overlooked for years:
light is the language your body uses to decide when to wake, when to slow down, and when to sleep.

And I had been speaking the wrong language for a long time.

When my sleep first began to falter, I didn't connect it to environment. I looked inward, stress, responsibility, pressure, all the usual suspects. I never asked myself whether my days were sending my nights off course. Yet every morning started the same way: a phone screen inches from my face, flooding my eyes with blue light before my feet even touched the floor. My brain wasn't waking up naturally. It was jolting into awareness like someone had thrown open the curtains in a dark room. And each time it happened, it shifted my internal rhythm just a little further out of alignment.

But mornings weren't the real problem. Evenings were.

My nights became an extension of my days, bright rooms, bright screens, bright thoughts. I treated late-night work as something admirable, proof I was pushing, grinding, getting ahead. I clicked through emails at 10PM with the same intensity I brought to the morning. I ended the day with my laptop open, the overhead lights blazing, the TV playing in the background, not because I needed it, but because stillness felt unnatural.

I didn't know then that every choice I made after sunset was sending a message to my nervous system: **"Stay awake. Stay alert. Something's happening."**

I wasn't giving my body the chance to downshift. I wasn't giving my brain the darkness it needed to release melatonin. I wasn't giving myself any cue, visual, emotional, or behavioral, that the day was ending. I'd built a life where nighttime looked and felt exactly like daytime, and my sleep paid the price long before I realized I was sabotaging myself.

People often assume sleep problems are personal flaws. They blame their discipline, their anxiety, their age, their genes. They don't realize that something as simple as how much light they see, and when they see it, can shift the entire architecture of their nights.

Our brains evolved to wind down as the world got darker. But now the world doesn't get dark. The sun may set, but our homes glow like midday. Screens shine directly into our eyes. Notifications flash. News scrolls. Work slides into the hours once reserved for calm. Every one of these inputs keeps the Behavioral System in "day mode," long past the point when the body is begging to slow down.

And because this shift happens slowly, nobody notices it.
You don't feel your internal clock drifting.
You don't feel melatonin suppression in real time.
You don't feel cortisol rising when it shouldn't.

You just know you're lying in bed wired and tired, wondering why your brain feels awake while every part of you wants rest.

Looking back, I can see how it happened to me. My days lost their shape. My nights lost their boundaries. There were no true transitions, no dimming, no slowing, no separation between effort and release. My behavior didn't prepare my body for sleep; it confused it.

What I didn't understand then, but understand now, is that the Behavioral System is the entry point for the entire sleep process. When your daily rhythm is steady, your nights follow that steadiness. When your behavior follows a clear pattern, your biology responds. But when your days become chaotic, when screens replace sunlight, when stimulation replaces stillness, when work follows you into the night, your body loses its sense of time.

It forgets when to shift.
It forgets when to soften.
It forgets when to sleep.

Not because it's broken,
but because the signals it depends on have been drowned out.

If you want to rebuild sleep, you start here, not with supplements, not with mantras, not with long routines you won't follow. You start by teaching your Behavioral System how to speak to your biology again. You start by restoring the rhythms your body once trusted without question.

Because sleep isn't just something that happens at night.
It begins with the way you live the day before.

Section 2: The Hidden Rhythms That Quietly Shape Your Nights

We like to think sleep is something that happens in isolation, a single event at the end of the day that lives separate from everything else we do. But sleep is never just about the night. It's a reflection of everything that comes before it, the choices we make, the pace we keep, the substances we consume, and the habits we repeat without thinking.

For most of my life, I didn't connect what I did at noon or five or eight o'clock with what happened at one in the morning. I thought a tough night was a tough night. I didn't realize it was a delayed consequence of the day.

Caffeine was the first culprit I never questioned. I told myself it was part of the grind. Morning tea, afternoon soda, evening stimulant if I still needed to push. I treated it like fuel, something I could pour in whenever my tank felt low. What I didn't see was the quiet residue it left behind, how it kept my nervous system humming long after the taste had faded. I assumed caffeine left my body when the energy faded, but that's not how it works. It lingers quietly, like an engine that won't fully shut off. You don't feel alert, but your brain does.

Looking back, I can see exactly how many nights were shaped by that simple mistake: thinking caffeine only affected me when I felt it. In reality, it was shaping my sleep hours later, sometimes deep into the night.

Alcohol was just as deceptive, even though I didn't drink much. It's easy to believe it helps you sleep because it makes you feel heavy, quiet, slow. On the surface it feels like relaxation, like the pressure slipping off your shoulders. But alcohol is a trickster. It knocks you out but doesn't keep you restored. I didn't know then that my "asleep" nights, after a drink or two, were fractured underneath the surface. I didn't know my brain was waking without waking, fighting to breathe, stuck in shallow sleep cycles that looked peaceful from the outside but left me drained by morning.

Even meals played a role I never expected. I used to eat late all the time, working through dinner, pushing tasks until I suddenly realized I was starving at nine or ten. I'd finally sit down to eat, only to feel heavy, restless, or wired later. I thought it was stress. It was actually biology. Digestion demands energy. It raises your temperature. It activates metabolic systems that directly compete with the processes needed for deep sleep. But because the consequences didn't appear immediately, I never even thought to make the connection.

Exercise followed the same pattern. Movement is supposed to help sleep, and it does, but timing matters. I used to push myself late at night, believing I was being disciplined, squeezing a workout in no matter what. I didn't realize that an elevated heart rate at 8:30 PM during a mixed martial arts class could sabotage my sleep at 11. I didn't realize that intensity at the wrong time can confuse the nervous system, tricking it into thinking the day is still active.

None of these behaviors seemed harmful. They were all just part of my rhythm, part of what life demanded, part of how I kept up. I wasn't careless. I wasn't reckless. I was living the way most high-performing people live: squeezing the day for everything it's worth.

But the body keeps score.

And the Behavioral System is always listening, always collecting signals, always preparing the night based on the day.

Looking back, the signs were subtle. A restless evening. A mind that wouldn't slow down. A body that felt too warm in bed. Nights where I fell asleep fast but woke up feeling like I hadn't slept at all. I didn't see these as consequences. I saw them as inconveniences, something to push through rather than something to understand.

What I didn't know then is something I understand now with absolute clarity: the Behavioral System is a translator, taking your daytime actions and sending messages to your nighttime biology.

Caffeine tells your body to stay vigilant.
Alcohol tells your body to disconnect instead of restore.
Late meals tell your body to digest, not rest.
Poorly timed exercise tells your body the day is still active.

None of these signals ruin sleep in one moment.
They shift it slowly.
They confuse it gradually.
They weaken its rhythm one choice at a time.

And the most dangerous part? You can live this way for months or years before the impact becomes too big to ignore.

For me, it wasn't one behavior that caused the crash. It was the accumulation. Caffeine layered on stress. Late meals layered on irregular rhythms. Evening light layered on emotional load. And together, those quiet misalignments built the framework for sleepless nights I didn't see coming.

Understanding this doesn't mean you have to live a rigid life or follow strict rules. It simply means acknowledging the reality most people never learn:

sleep is shaped long before the night begins.

Once you see the connection, you can change it.
And once you change it, sleep begins to return in ways that feel almost inevitable.

Section 3: Work Cycles, Travel, and Social Habits, The Invisible Disruptors

There are parts of life that disrupt sleep so subtly that you don't recognize their impact until you're already in trouble. Work schedules. Travel. Social obligations. The constant negotiations you make with your time in order to keep up with everything and everyone. These aren't "bad habits." They're the markers of a modern life, especially for high performers, people who carry more than most, who lead, who build, who manage teams, who support families, who push forward even when the world feels heavy.

For years, my work cycles ran my life. I told myself it was temporary, just a season, just a deadline, just a busy stretch. I lived in a pattern of long days, late nights, and early mornings, convincing myself this was the only way to meet the goals I'd set. I didn't realize that this pattern itself, constant expansion, no boundaries, no predictable end to the day, was quietly eroding the scaffolding sleep depends on.

There were stretches where I'd stop working physically, but mentally I stayed in motion. Even after shutting my laptop, my brain stayed in strategy mode, still carrying the weight of unfinished decisions. Work didn't end at the end of the day; it followed me into the evening and often into bed. And when the mind stays in "day mode," the body follows. Sleep doesn't come to a system that never truly stops working.

Travel made everything worse. I treated travel as a minor inconvenience, something you push through, time zones, long drives, airport stress, hotel beds, new environments. You adjust. You adapt. You get the job done. But your body doesn't adapt as easily as your mind does. Each time you travel, you break your rhythm. You shift your eating schedule, your exposure to light, your sense of routine. You sleep in unfamiliar rooms where your brain automatically becomes more alert, scanning for safety the way humans have done for thousands of years.

It doesn't matter how comfortable the hotel is.
It's not home.
And your body knows the difference.

Social habits play their own quiet role. Most of us don't realize that late dinners, late conversations, staying out longer than planned, saying yes to obligations that stretch into the night, these things reshape the behavioral cues your body relies on. You tell yourself it's just one evening. But one evening becomes many. Nights get later. Meals shift. Bedtime pushes back. You start drifting away from consistency without noticing.

And because everyone around you is doing the same, staying up late, answering messages at all hours, saying they're tired but pushing through, you don't see these choices as harmful. You see them as normal.

But normal and natural are not the same.

Normal is the culture we've built.
Natural is the rhythm we were designed for.
Sleep depends on the natural rhythm, not the cultural one.

The most dangerous part about work cycles, travel, and social habits is that none of them feel extreme. They don't feel like sabotage. They feel inevitable, like part of the life you've built. You don't realize you're stretching yourself thin because you're still performing. You're still meeting expectations. You're still keeping up. And as long as you can keep up, you believe everything is fine.

But the Behavioral System tells a different story.

It keeps score.
It notices irregularity.
It senses unpredictability.
It recognizes when there is no true "end" to the day.

And once it loses trust in your routine, it stops preparing for sleep the way it once did. You can feel it when this shift begins, not through insomnia at first, but through subtle changes: nights where you feel slightly out of sync, mornings where you wake up a little heavier, evenings where you can't quite slow down even though you're tired.

I used to believe I could outrun these patterns. That discipline would fix everything. That drive and accomplishment would override the effects of long days, late nights, cross-country flights, and unpredictable schedules. But sleep is not something you can overpower. It's something you support.

The truth is simple:
Most people don't lose sleep because they're weak.
They lose sleep because their lives no longer follow a rhythm their body understands.

Work cycles stretch the day.
Travel breaks the cues.
Social habits shift the timing.
And sleep, obedient, delicate, ancient, tries to adapt until it can't anymore.

Once you understand this, you begin to see your daily life differently. You stop assuming you're the problem. You start recognizing that your sleep is only reflecting the shape of your days.

And that's the good news:
When you reshape the day, the night begins to repair itself.

Section 4: The Patterns You Don't Notice… Until They Break You

The most dangerous behaviors for sleep are never the dramatic ones. They're the quiet habits you repeat without thinking, habits so familiar, so baked into your rhythm, that you stop seeing them as choices. They become the background noise of life, subtle enough to ignore but powerful enough to destabilize an entire sleep system.

Most people imagine their sleep problems come from something obvious: a bad night, a stressful week, a big project, an argument, a deadline. But in truth, the collapse usually comes from the tiny patterns that slip beneath awareness. They accumulate. Layer by layer. And long before you're lying awake at 2AM wondering what happened to you, those patterns have already been shaping your nights.

I know this because I lived inside those patterns for years before I ever recognized them for what they were.

The Quiet Drift Into Overdrive

For me, it started with something as simple as shortening the space between activities. I'd finish a call and immediately start another. Leave a meeting and jump straight into the next task. Eat lunch at my desk. Return messages while walking to the car. When the day ended, it didn't really end, my mind stayed in motion, carrying the pace of the day into the night like momentum I couldn't slow.

Nothing about it looked unhealthy from the outside. This was normal life for most high performers I knew. But the body keeps score, even when you believe you're outsmarting it.

Your nervous system is built around transitions, tiny downshifts that tell the body the day is moving toward rest. When those micro-pauses disappear, your brain never receives the signal to slow down. Instead, it adapts to the rhythm you force on it. It learns speed. It learns urgency. It learns momentum. And what you practice all day becomes the state you bring into bed.

The Unseen Stimulants of a Modern Life

There were other patterns, too, small decisions that felt harmless but quietly rewired the system:

Scrolling during the last ten minutes before bed.
Telling myself I just needed to "get ahead" by checking one more email.
Switching on a bright kitchen light late at night without thinking.
Leaving a TV show playing in the background because the silence felt too sharp.
Jumping into intense conversations after 9PM because that's when the world slows enough for people to talk deeply.

None of these actions seemed significant. They were routine, even comforting in their familiarity. But they kept my mind looking outward instead of inward, searching instead of softening, reacting instead of releasing.

At the time, I didn't recognize how these small behaviors stacked on top of one another. I didn't see that they were training my nervous system to stay alert even when I was exhausted. I didn't connect these rituals to the nights I felt wired for no reason, or the mornings that felt foggy even after long hours in bed.

But the body noticed.
The body always notices.

The False Calm of Constant Busyness

One of the most deceptive patterns is using busyness as a buffer against rest.
A lot of people do this without realizing it. I certainly did.

Being busy feels productive. It feels like control. It feels like momentum. And
when you're wired to lead, to make things happen, to hold the weight of
others, busyness becomes a kind of self-protection. It keeps your mind from
drifting into the deeper, quieter spaces where unresolved thoughts live.

The trouble is that busyness doesn't dissolve the emotional load, it only delays
it. And when the day finally ends, that backlog hits your mind all at once. Not
because something new happened, but because everything you didn't process
finally has room to surface.

People interpret this flood as anxiety or rumination. They assume something
is wrong with their mind. But often, it's simply the cost of never giving it
space during the day.

When Familiar Habits Become Invisible Sabotage

Patterns like:

- rushing through evenings

- eating dinner late

- working under bright lights

- multitasking until bedtime

- treating wind-down time as optional

…don't look harmful. But they train your system into a state that is the exact
opposite of what sleep requires.

That mismatch creates a nightly battle:
your biology trying to slow down while your behaviors keep speeding up.

For me, this realization didn't come in a dramatic moment. It arrived slowly, through observation, through finally noticing how much of my life was lived in forward motion. I began to see how rarely I allowed myself to switch gears, how little space there was between my day and my night, how automatic my habits had become.

And once you see it, you can't unsee it.

The Truth About Subtle Sabotage

The behavioral system rarely collapses suddenly.
It erodes.

Each small pattern, on its own, changes nothing.
But together, over months and years, they build an internal environment where sleep can't find its way in.

This isn't about blame.
It's about awareness.

Because once you understand that the smallest habits carry the greatest weight, you finally regain control. You can create space where there was none. You can build transitions where life once moved in a single unbroken stream. You can retrain the body to recognize the difference between day and night.

You can stop sabotaging sleep without ever intending to.

And that's the beginning of restoring the Behavioral System, by acknowledging that sleep is built long before you get into bed, through the tiny choices you make without noticing.

Section 5: How a Life Built on Adrenaline Weakens Sleep

There are people who drift through life at a comfortable pace, and then there are people like us, the ones who run on momentum, who carry responsibility like it's welded to our shoulders, who move quickly because slowing down has never felt like an option.

For years, I didn't just live with adrenaline. I lived *on* it. It was the fuel behind my long days, the force that pushed me through deadlines, travel, stress, and everything I believed I had to carry without breaking. Adrenaline sharpened me. It made me effective. It made me a provider, a leader, a protector.

It also quietly dismantled my ability to sleep.

What I didn't understand then, and what most people never connect, is that adrenaline is not just a feeling. It's a physiological state. Once it becomes your default, your body stops remembering how to enter any other one.

I used to think exhaustion meant I was doing something right. That tension meant I was focused. That pushing through meant I was strong. I'd wake up already moving, handle a dozen things before breakfast, and plow through the day without ever checking in with myself. My mind was active from the moment I opened my eyes to the moment I finally shut them at night. That pace didn't feel extreme. It felt necessary.

But adrenaline has a cost. A quiet cost.

The body isn't designed to live in "go mode" indefinitely. It's built for cycles, activation, then recovery. Movement, then stillness. Effort, then rest. When adrenaline becomes the foundation of your day, those cycles disappear. You stay charged long after the work ends. You stay alert long after the danger passes. You stay wired even when you're exhausted.

It took me years to realize that adrenaline is a thief. It steals the ability to transition. It makes your internal state rigid, unable to soften or slow. Adrenaline teaches your nervous system one message repeatedly: **stay ready.**

And a body that is trained to stay ready never fully sleeps.

It doesn't matter how tired you are.
It doesn't matter how badly you want rest.
It doesn't matter how many routines, supplements, or hacks you try.

If your days are built on adrenaline, your nights will be built on resistance.

I saw it come to life in subtle ways long before my sleep collapsed:

Nights where I lay in bed feeling tired but *charged*, like my body was buzzing with leftover electricity. Mornings where I woke up already tense, already thinking about the next ten steps before I even left the pillow. Days when even small problems felt urgent because my system treated everything as a trigger.

That wasn't personality.
It wasn't drive.
It wasn't discipline.

It was adrenaline doing what adrenaline does, keeping me upright while quietly burning through the resources my sleep would later need.

The truth is, many high performers mistake adrenaline for energy. For motivation. For capability. But adrenaline isn't energy you *have*, it's energy you *borrow*. It gives you a surge now and sends the bill later. And the bill is always paid at night.

You can't rest deeply with adrenaline in your bloodstream. You can't cycle into restorative sleep when your body is bracing for impact. Adrenaline doesn't allow surrender. It doesn't allow vulnerability. It doesn't allow the nervous system to shift into the slow rhythms required for true restoration.

People often tell me, "I'm exhausted, but the moment I lie down, I'm wide awake."
Of course they are.
They've lived the entire day in a mode that teaches the body the opposite of sleep.

My own turning point came when I finally realized this: I didn't have a sleep problem. I had an adrenaline lifestyle. And as long as my days stayed wired, my nights never stood a chance.

Fixing sleep didn't begin with bedtime routines. It began with unwinding a life built on urgency, learning how to transition, how to decelerate, how to build days that didn't require me to run hot from morning until night.

Adrenaline had been the engine of my success.
It was also the architect of my downfall.

And until I saw that clearly, nothing changed.

This chapter exists because most people struggling with sleep aren't failing at night. They're living in a way during the day that makes healthy nights impossible.

Sleep begins long before your head reaches the pillow.
It begins the moment you wake up,
in the pace you choose,
the pressure you carry,
the urgency you feed,
and the nervous system you build hour by hour.

When your days stop running on adrenaline, your nights can finally return to what they were designed to be: a place of true restoration, not recovery from the damage the day inflicted.

Chapter 5: The Biological System

Section 1: Circadian Rhythm Timing

The first time my sleep truly began to break down, I didn't recognize it as
biology. I blamed stress, workload, habits, anything but the truth. Because
when you're used to being strong, you assume every problem is a problem
you can outwork. But sleep doesn't bend to effort. It bends to rhythm. And
the rhythm inside your body, the circadian rhythm, was quietly steering
everything long before you ever realized something was off.

We like to think we control our days. That we choose when we're tired, when
we're alert, when we're hungry, when we're ready to shut down. But the truth
is much simpler and far more humbling: your circadian rhythm controls all of
it. You live inside its timing whether you know it or not. And when that
timing drifts, sleep becomes one of the first casualties.

For most of human history, this internal clock was perfectly synced to the
world around us. Sunrise told the brain to wake. Sunset signaled the slow
descent into rest. Our biology took cues from nature, light, temperature,
darkness, and aligned itself accordingly. We didn't have to think about sleep
because the environment handled it for us.

Then modern life arrived.

Lights. Screens. Late nights. Early mornings. Long commutes. Jet lag. Shift
work. Caffeine at all hours. Meals whenever we can fit them in. Work that
follows us home. Stress that never ends. A schedule that doesn't resemble
anything our biology evolved for.

Little by little, our internal clock stops matching the world outside us, or the
lives we actually lead. And when the clock drifts, everything drifts.

For me, it showed up quietly at first. I'd feel alert late into the evening,
convinced I was just a "night person." I'd get a second wind at exactly the
time I should've been winding down. My mornings felt heavier, slower, as if
waking required something more than sleep could give. I pushed through it,
assuming I'd "catch up" eventually. I never did.

Because you can't catch up to a clock that's no longer in sync.

That's what circadian misalignment feels like:
nights where you're tired but unable to drop,
mornings where you're awake but not restored,
days where energy comes at all the wrong times.

The body becomes confused. Melatonin releases too late or too early. Cortisol spikes at the wrong moment. Temperature cycles shift. Digestion drifts. Hormones fire off-pattern. And the person living in that body starts to believe something is wrong with *them* instead of the system that's breaking beneath the surface.

I spent years thinking my sleep issues were mental. Emotional. Stress-induced. And while those played a part, the deeper truth was simpler: the rhythm inside my body was no longer matching the life I was living. My brain thought night was day and day was night. It was trying to cycle naturally in a world that refused to slow down enough to let it.

Circadian misalignment isn't dramatic. It's not loud. It doesn't collapse overnight. It shifts in degrees, a subtle slide that pulls your sleep further from its natural anchor. And because it happens gradually, you blame everything except biology.

If you've ever found yourself tired at the wrong times, wired when you want rest, alert long after the lights go off, or dragging yourself through mornings that feel heavier than they should, you've felt it. It's not laziness. Not lack of discipline. Not a broken brain. It's simply a rhythm that's been knocked off course.

And here's the part most people never hear:
Circadian misalignment is reversible.
But only when you understand what's really happening.

Your sleep struggles didn't emerge from nowhere. They emerged from timing, timing that was quietly altered by the world you move through, the pace you live at, and the habits you never realized were signaling your biology to shift.

This chapter exists to bring you back into rhythm, not through willpower, but through alignment. Because once your clock resets, your nights begin to restore themselves. Effortlessly. Naturally. Predictably.

Sleep doesn't just depend on biology. It begins with it.

Section 2: Cortisol–Melatonin Patterns

If the circadian rhythm is your body's clock, then cortisol and melatonin are the gears that make that clock move. They rise and fall in a dance so precise that your sleep depends on it. When they move in harmony, nights feel peaceful and predictable. When they collide or trade places, sleep becomes a fight you can't win, no matter how exhausted you are.

For a long time, I didn't know anything about cortisol or melatonin beyond the basics everyone repeats online. "Melatonin helps you sleep." "Cortisol wakes you up." Simple. Clean. Easy to understand. Except it's far more complicated, and far more fragile, than that.

Your body is designed to follow a natural pattern:

Cortisol rises in the morning, steadily lifting your alertness, sharpening your focus, helping you feel ready for the day.
Melatonin rises at night, signaling the brain that it's time to wind down, release tension, lower temperature, and drift into rest.

The two are supposed to sit on opposite ends of a seesaw. When one rises, the other falls. That balance is what creates deep, restorative sleep.

But modern life doesn't respect that balance.

Stress pushes cortisol higher than it should be.
Late-night screens delay melatonin.
Irregular routines confuse the entire system.
And slowly, quietly, the seesaw stops working.

I didn't notice it at first.
I just knew that when night came, I wasn't calming the way I should. I'd lie down tired but feel a kind of internal hum, like my body was idling too high. It wasn't dramatic. It didn't feel like panic. It just felt… wrong. As if my mind and body were on two different wavelengths.

That hum, I later learned, was cortisol, the hormone meant to carry me through the morning, showing up at night instead.

People think cortisol is the "stress hormone," but it's really the "alertness hormone," the signal that tells your body it's time to be awake, aware, ready. When that signal fires at night, sleep becomes nearly impossible. Your mind races. Your body tenses. Your thoughts sharpen instead of soften. You feel wired and tired at the same time, the worst combination a person can live inside.

And melatonin? It doesn't stand a chance when cortisol is crowding the system.

Here's the part most people never hear:
Your body doesn't release melatonin just because you're tired.
It releases melatonin because your environment and routines tell it to.

Darkness.
Predictability.
Warmth dropping.
Silence.
Simplicity.

These are the cues that cue melatonin.
None of which exist in modern life unless you intentionally create them.

For years, my patterns worked against me.
Late-night emails.
Bright screens.
Constant deadlines.
Stress that followed me into every evening.
A mind conditioned to stay alert long after the day ended.

Cortisol crept into the night.
Melatonin slid later and later.
And I mistook the entire cycle for "stress," never realizing my hormones had swapped places entirely.

It's a strange feeling, to be desperate for rest while your body is signaling wakefulness. You feel betrayed by your own biology. But hormones aren't malicious. They're obedient. They respond to whatever pattern you repeatedly expose them to.

The truth is simple:
Your body wasn't failing you.
It was responding perfectly to an imperfect environment.

High cortisol at night doesn't mean you're weak.
Low melatonin at bedtime doesn't mean you're broken.
It means your system is trying to adapt to the pace and pressure of your life.

And here's the most important piece:
The system can be reset.

Once cortisol returns to the morning, once melatonin rises naturally in the evening, once the seesaw begins to balance again, sleep stops feeling like an uphill battle. It becomes automatic, because biology is finally working with you instead of against you.

This section of the book isn't just about understanding hormones.
It's about reclaiming the rhythm that stress, screens, and modern life quietly took from you.

Because sleep doesn't return through force.
It returns when cortisol and melatonin remember their roles, and your life is finally aligned enough for them to play their part.

Section 3: Temperature Regulation

Most people never think about temperature when they think about sleep. It sounds too simple, too small, too basic to matter. The truth is the opposite: temperature is one of the most powerful biological levers in the entire sleep system, and when it's off, even slightly, your body can't enter deep rest.

Real sleep requires a drop in core body temperature.
Not a preference. Not a comfort issue.
A biological necessity.

Your internal thermostat, the system that controls your core heat, is directly tied to the parts of your brain responsible for initiating and maintaining sleep. When that temperature begins to fall in the evening, it sends a message through your nervous system:

"It's nighttime. It's safe. You can let go."

Without that drop, the signal never completes.

I didn't know any of this during the years my sleep was slipping. I just knew something felt wrong. I'd lie there feeling restless in a way I couldn't explain. Not mentally restless, physically. Like my body wanted to sink into the mattress but couldn't. My chest felt warm, my face felt hot, my legs kept shifting, and I'd drift in and out without ever reaching that heavy, grounded calm that deep sleep brings.

Back then, I blamed everything *except* temperature.
Stress.
Workload.
Age.
Overthinking.
Responsibility.
Life.

Temperature felt too trivial to matter.

But it wasn't trivial. It was central.

Every night, my body was trying to cool itself enough to sleep, and I was unknowingly working against it. Late workouts. Hot showers. Eating too close to bedtime. Too many blankets. A room that was just a couple degrees warmer than ideal. Each one raised my core temperature just enough to disrupt the entire process.

And the body doesn't negotiate on this.
If your temperature stays even 1–2 degrees too high, your brain simply won't drop into deep sleep. You stay hovering on the surface, drifting, dozing, waking, never sinking.

There's another layer to this:
Stress raises temperature.
Inflammation raises temperature.
Adrenaline raises temperature.
Cortisol raises temperature.
A wired nervous system heats the body from the inside out.

People think they're tossing and turning because they're anxious. Sometimes they're tossing and turning because their core hasn't cooled enough to let them rest.

I can remember nights where I wasn't thinking about anything at all, no spiraling mind, no racing thoughts, just this uncomfortable sense of internal heat. My body felt like it was stuck in "day mode," even though the clock said night. I'd flip the blanket off, pull it back on, stick a leg out, try to breathe slower, try to find a position that didn't feel suffocating.

It never clicked.
Not then.

Because nobody teaches us that thermal regulation isn't optional.
It's part of the biological script of sleep.

In the hours before natural bedtime, your core temperature is supposed to drop. That drop is one of the primary triggers for melatonin release. When you move through life in ways that keep your temperature elevated, late meals, screens, stress, intense evening exercise, your body doesn't reach the cooling threshold.

And the worst part?
When temperature doesn't drop, your sleep fragments.

You wake repeatedly.
You dream less vividly.
You hover in light sleep.
You wake feeling unrefreshed.
Your heart rate stays elevated.
Your breath stays shallow.
Your brain never dips into deep, restorative cycles.

When I finally learned how tightly sleep is tied to body temperature, everything made sense. All the nights where I felt internally "revved." All the early wake-ups where my chest felt hot. All the mornings where I woke feeling like I'd barely slept even though I was unconscious for hours.

Temperature wasn't a comfort issue.
It was a biological signal my body wasn't receiving.

Once I began adjusting my environment, cooler air, lighter bedding, consistent evening routines, the shift was dramatic. Not immediate, but unmistakable. My body finally had the conditions it needed to start the descent into sleep again. The nights weren't perfect, but they were no longer a battle. My biology wasn't fighting itself.

This is one of the most important things people must understand:
Your body is always communicating with you.
Temperature is one of its clearest messages.

When it cools, sleep comes.
When it stays warm, sleep resists.

This is not weakness.
This is not "bad sleep."
This is biology doing exactly what biology does, responding to the conditions it's given.

And for the first time, you can give it the conditions it's been missing.

Section 4: Digestion + Metabolic Load

There's a moment late in the evening, usually somewhere between the last emails, the last dishes, the last scroll through your phone, when the day finally feels like it should be over. Your mind says, *"I'm done."* Your body says, *"I'm tired."*
But if you've eaten too late, or too heavily, or too irregularly, there's another part of you that isn't anywhere near finished: your digestive system.

Most people never consider digestion as part of their sleep equation.
They think of food as fuel, meals as schedule blocks, and eating as a daily necessity that has nothing to do with nighttime physiology. But the truth is simple and unavoidable:

If your digestion is active, restorative sleep is not.

Your digestive system is one of the most energy-demanding systems in your entire body. It requires focus, blood flow, metabolic activation, temperature increases, all signals that are the opposite of what your sleep system needs.

Restoration requires stillness.
Digestion requires activation.
When these two collide, sleep loses every time.

For years, I ignored this.
Late dinners.
Heavy meals after long days.
Snacks in front of the TV as I tried to "wind down."
Grabbing food between work calls.
Eating on travel schedules that made no sense for my biology.

If I was hungry, I ate.
If I was stressed, I ate.
If I was rushing, I ate whatever was fastest.
And if I was exhausted and finally catching my breath at 9 or 10 PM, well,
that became dinnertime.

I didn't see the pattern at first.
I just knew my nights felt uneasy, my sleep fragmented, my chest tight, and
my mornings drained. I assumed it was stress. Or pace. Or the weight I was
carrying. And yes, those were part of it, but so was the simple fact that my
digestion was still in high gear long after I needed it to be silent.

Food changes everything about your internal environment.
It raises core temperature.
It elevates heart rate.
It activates insulin.
It signals your body to stay awake and process.
It pulls blood flow toward the stomach and away from the brain regions that
regulate deep sleep.

Even light meals can keep the system humming just enough to delay the
transition into rest.

But heavy meals?
High fat?
Late-night sugar?
Alcohol mixed with meals?
These don't just disturb sleep, they can derail it entirely.

What most people call "anxiety at night" is often metabolic:
• a glucose drop
• a cortisol spike
• an adrenaline jolt triggered by unstable blood sugar
• a digestive system straining to process food long after the body wants to shut down

I lived that for months without knowing.
There were nights I'd wake at 2 or 3 AM heartbeat climbing, mind instantly alert, chest feeling warm, convinced my thoughts had jolted me awake.
But it wasn't always thoughts.
It was biology.

Your body is not designed to multitask sleep and digestion.
When push comes to shove, the body chooses survival.
Digestion ranks higher on the priority list than deep sleep.

You can be unconscious without being rested, and digestion is one of the fastest ways to create that divide.

There's a deeper truth to this, one I didn't understand until much later:
When your days lack rhythm, your eating lacks rhythm.
And when your eating lacks rhythm, your sleep loses timing.

Your circadian system depends on predictable metabolic cues:
• when you eat
• how heavily you eat
• how late you eat
• how often you eat

These cues help your internal clock decide when to release melatonin, when to lower core temperature, when to shift into parasympathetic calm.

If those cues are chaotic, your sleep cycles become chaotic too.

I learned the hard way that food isn't just fuel, it's instruction.
Every meal gives your body a message.
Late-night meals send the wrong ones.

•

Once I started aligning my eating with what my biology actually needed, lighter evenings, consistent timing, more space between dinner and bed, sleep didn't instantly become perfect, but it became possible again.
My nights stopped feeling like internal battles.
My wake-ups became softer, fewer, easier to move past.
My mornings didn't feel like punishment.

Digestion doesn't get a lot of attention in sleep conversations.
But this is one of the most overlooked truths in the entire field:

Your sleep can only deepen to the level your metabolism is willing to allow.

If you give your body the space to process food when the sun is still up, it will give you the space to sleep when the night comes.

Sleep is a biological rhythm.
Digestion is a biological rhythm.
They must respect each other.
If they don't, one of them collapses.
And for millions of people, including me at one point, sleep is the one that breaks first.

Section 5: Hormonal and Age-Related Shifts

You can go most of your early life without giving a single thought to hormones. When you're young, your biology works in the background like a perfect machine, quiet, reliable, invisible. You don't think about cortisol cycles or melatonin timing or testosterone levels or thyroid activity. You don't think about how your body generates energy, regulates temperature, repairs tissue, or keeps your metabolism balanced.

You just live.
And sleep simply shows up.

But as you move into your 30s, 40s, and beyond, the internal landscape begins to shift in ways most people don't recognize until it's already affecting their nights. The machinery still works, but not automatically, and not without influence from stress, lifestyle, and age. The rhythms that once took care of themselves now need more support, more structure, more consistency.

For me, this shift wasn't dramatic, it was subtle. A slow drift. A feeling that something was "off," even though my days looked the same. I chalked it up to busyness or pressure or ambition. It took years before I understood that part of what I was fighting wasn't just my habits or my environment, it was hormones that had quietly begun to operate on new terms.

Cortisol is often the first to change.
When you're young, cortisol rises in the morning like a switch turning on. It gives you energy, motivation, alertness. Then it drops through the day, preparing your body for rest. But stress, especially chronic stress, shifts that curve. If your days become a string of unresolved pressures, late nights, and nonstop demands, your body starts releasing cortisol at inconsistent times.

Before long, evening becomes the new morning.
You feel wired at night when you're supposed to be winding down.
You feel heavy and slow when you wake up.

You don't blame cortisol.
You blame yourself.

Melatonin shifts next.
It's a hormone of darkness and rhythm, one that depends on predictable cues: light fading, temperature dropping, schedules stabilizing. But if your nights are bright and your routines unpredictable, your melatonin release doesn't know when to begin. For years, I didn't even consider this. I just assumed I was a "night person," someone who liked working late, someone whose mind didn't settle until the world went quiet.

But my biology wasn't built that way.
My habits made it that way.

Then there's testosterone, something most men avoid talking about but silently worry over when sleep falls apart. Testosterone supports energy, mood regulation, motivation, and even the depth of slow-wave sleep. As levels drop with age, or drop faster because of stress, poor sleep, or overtraining, you feel it long before you admit it. Recovery slows. Your resilience dips. Emotional volatility rises. Nights feel lighter, more fragile.

You tell yourself you're overwhelmed.
Or getting older.
Or "just tired."
But the truth is often simpler:
Your biology is working with fewer resources.

Thyroid function plays its role too, especially in people who operate at high speed. When the thyroid slows, even slightly, everything becomes heavier, energy, mood, digestion, and sleep. When it speeds up, sleep becomes restless and choppy. Most people never consider the thyroid until years into their struggle. I didn't either. I mistook the signs for stress, because stress was familiar and easier to blame.

Then there's the metabolic shift that happens as you age.
Your body becomes less forgiving, of late meals, irregular sleep, stimulants, alcohol, long work cycles. In your twenties, you can abuse your rhythms and bounce back. By your forties, your biology asks for respect, with or without your permission.

But here's the part that matters most:
Hormonal changes don't cause sleep issues on their own.
They magnify whatever is already out of alignment.

If your behavioral system is chaotic, hormonal shifts make it feel overwhelming.
If your emotional system is overloaded, hormonal shifts amplify the tension.
If your biological system is drifting, hormonal shifts push it further.

This is where so many people misinterpret what's happening. When they feel their energy dip or their patience thin or their sleep lighten, they assume age is to blame. They think this is simply what getting older feels like. But age isn't the enemy, it's the amplifier. It takes the patterns you've lived with for years and reveals their consequences more clearly.

I had to learn this too.
Not in a moment, but over many nights, many mornings, many small realizations that finally connected into a larger truth:

Your hormones don't fail you.
They follow you.

They mirror your pace.
Your habits.
Your stress load.
Your sleep patterns.
Your alignment, or misalignment.

And the moment you begin repairing the systems around them, they respond. Sometimes surprisingly quickly. Sometimes gradually and quietly. But they respond.

That's the beauty of the biological system:
It is not rigid.
It is not doomed.
It is not fixed in decline.

It adapts.
It recalibrates.
It heals.

Once you understand the role hormones play, you stop blaming yourself. You stop fearing age. You stop believing sleep is something slipping through your fingers. Instead, you start seeing it as a system waiting for the right conditions to do what it's always been capable of.

And that's where the real work, and the real relief, begins.

Section 6: Breathing, Airway Collapse, and CPAP

Most people think of sleep as something that happens in the mind, thoughts slowing, emotions settling, consciousness dimming. But some of the most powerful forces shaping your nights live deeper, in parts of the body you rarely think about when you're awake. Breathing is one of them. In fact, for millions of people, disrupted breathing is the silent engine behind years of unexplained exhaustion, nighttime panic, and mornings that feel like they never begin cleanly.

It took me far too long to learn this.

When my sleep first began to unravel, I assumed it was stress, overwork, responsibility, anything but physiology. Even when I woke up with my heart pounding, or gasping for air, or feeling like my chest was too tight to settle, I didn't connect the dots. I told myself I was overwhelmed. I told myself I needed better routines. I told myself this was part of the grind.

But breathing, especially at night, is not something you can out-discipline.
You can fight a wandering mind.
You can push through fatigue.
You can argue with your thoughts.
But you can't force your airway to stay open with willpower.

The airway is a delicate structure. When you fall asleep, muscles relax. The tongue shifts. The jaw settles. For most people, everything stays open enough for air to move freely. But for others, the airway narrows just enough that breathing becomes inconsistent. Sometimes it's restless snoring. Sometimes it's shallow breaths interrupted by tiny gasps. And sometimes, without realizing it, breathing stops altogether, for a few seconds, tens of seconds, or longer.

This is sleep-disordered breathing.
Often apnea.
Often undiagnosed.
Often the real cause behind years of misery.

Night after night, your brain senses the oxygen drop and jolts you awake, sometimes fully, sometimes just enough to disrupt the sleep cycle. You don't remember these micro-awakenings, but your body does. It wakes feeling as though you fought something all night long.

That's exactly what happened to me.

At first, it came in whispers: waking with a dry mouth, a tight chest, a sudden jerk as if falling from a height. I wrote it off as stress. Then came nights where I'd wake in the dark struggling for air, convinced something emotional was happening when something physical was happening instead. I felt exhausted in ways that didn't match my schedule. No amount of discipline could touch it. No amount of routine could fix it.

Because the problem wasn't in my habits.
It was in my airway.

There's a specific frustration that comes with this phase, the sense that your mind is doing everything right while your body is quietly failing at something as primitive as breathing. You lie there in the dark, tired but wired, heavy but restless, drifting but never falling. You feel like something inside you is misfiring, but you can't see it. You can't measure it. You can't control it. And because the symptoms show up as exhaustion, fog, irritability, or nighttime anxiety, you blame yourself.

Millions do.

It wasn't until I went through a sleep evaluation that the truth surfaced:
my airway wasn't staying open at night.
My oxygen dropped.
My brain repeatedly woke me to save my life.
And I had been calling that "insomnia."

That's the tragedy of sleep-disordered breathing, it hides inside symptoms people mislabel for years. Call it stress. Call it anxiety. Call it overthinking. Call it aging. Call it anything but what it actually is.

And when the diagnosis comes, when someone finally names what's been happening, people often feel two things at once: validation and dread. Validation because the mystery finally has a cause. Dread because the solution, for many, is a CPAP machine.

That was my reaction too.

There's a humbling moment when you see that machine for the first time, the mask, the hose, the pressure. It feels clinical, intrusive, like a symbol of something you never imagined needing. But what I learned is that CPAP is less a burden and more a bridge. It's the moment your body starts getting oxygen again. The moment your brain stops waking in panic. The moment sleep becomes more than unconsciousness, it becomes recovery.

The first nights were strange.
The first mornings were unfamiliar.
But slowly, something shifted.

For the first time in years, I woke up with a clarity I didn't recognize. The heaviness that sat in my chest began to lift. The grogginess that followed me into every morning began to fade. The fatigue that no amount of mindset work could touch finally began to break. It was like discovering a version of myself I'd forgotten was possible.

Not because the machine fixed me.
But because my biology finally had a chance to do what it had been trying to do all along: breathe, restore, recover.

That's the deeper lesson here:
Sleep is not just about drifting off.
It's about everything your body must do to keep you alive while you're down. If breathing fails, the whole system collapses.

That's why so many people who feel stuck in endless cycles of exhaustion, nighttime panic, or "mystery insomnia" are actually fighting oxygen deprivation they can't see. It's why the mind feels wired. Why the heart races. Why the nights feel unpredictable. Why the mornings feel heavy. It's why no sleep hack, meditation app, or routine can fix what's fundamentally physical.

You can't out-think a blocked airway.
You can only diagnose it.
And then support it.

Once you do, everything else, the emotional work, the behavioral changes, the routines and rhythms, finally has something solid to rest on.

Your body finally stops fighting for air.
And can finally fight for sleep.

Section 7: What Chronic Stress Did Inside Your Body

There's a moment, usually years into the struggle, when people look at their restless nights and wonder, *"How did it get this bad? How did my body fall so far out of sync?"*
The truth is, it didn't happen suddenly. It happened slowly, through a kind of internal wear-and-tear that builds quietly beneath the surface until the body can no longer hide it.

Chronic stress doesn't just make you feel overwhelmed.
It alters the machinery of your biology.

At first, stress shows up in ways you can sense: tension, irritability, a racing mind. But when it goes on long enough, when the body is asked to perform for months or years without real recovery, stress begins to imprint itself into deeper systems: your hormones, your temperature regulation, your digestion, your breathing, your blood sugar, your cardiovascular rhythm. It becomes embedded, structural.

I didn't understand this during the early stages of my own collapse. Like most people who operate at full speed, I believed stress was something you could outrun or out-work. If I just pushed a little harder or stayed focused or stayed disciplined, I assumed my body would fall in line.

But biology doesn't care about determination.
It responds only to load.

And I had been loading my system beyond capacity for years.

At some point, long before the sleepless nights fully took hold, my stress had shifted from a temporary state into a chronic condition. I didn't notice it happening. It didn't announce itself. It didn't derail my days. It simply lived in the background, tightening small screws inside my body one at a time.

Here's what chronic stress does when it stays too long:

It rewires your cortisol rhythm.

Cortisol is supposed to peak in the morning and fall at night. Under chronic stress, that curve inverts. You wake sluggish and crash late, only to feel wired when you should be winding down. Over time, the body forgets when "day" is supposed to start and when "night" is supposed to end.

That's exactly what happened to me, I would drag myself through mornings and then somehow hit a second wind when the sun went down. It felt like a productivity boost. It was actually physiological misalignment.

It disrupts your sleep-wake timing.

Stress interferes with the slow cascade of internal signals that normally prepare your body for sleep: cooling temperature, lowering cortisol, rising melatonin, stabilizing heart rate. When those cues get scrambled, sleep becomes unpredictable. Some nights you fall asleep easily. Some nights you can't. Some nights you wake in a jolt for no reason.

That unpredictability does more damage than a single bad night ever could.

It changes your internal temperature control.

Most people don't realize how crucial temperature is to sleep. Your body must drop a degree or two internally before it can drift off. Chronic stress interferes with that drop. The system stays warm, activated, ready. You lie in bed feeling restless, tossing sheets aside, trying to get comfortable when the truth is simple: your body never got the signal to cool.

Been there. For months, I couldn't find a position that felt "right." I didn't know then that it wasn't the bed. It was me, stuck in a heat pattern caused by stress.

It destabilizes blood sugar.

Stress raises glucose. Elevated glucose causes nighttime spikes and crashes. Crashes trigger adrenaline. Adrenaline wakes you, heart pounding, mind racing, confused about why you're suddenly alert. Many people think that moment is anxiety. Often, it's biology.

Those abrupt 2 or 3 AM wake-ups I kept having?
They weren't worry.
They were chemistry.

It keeps the sympathetic nervous system in charge.

The sympathetic system is your "go" mode.
The parasympathetic system is your "rest" mode.
Chronic stress keeps the sympathetic system running by default. That means your heart rate stays a little higher, your muscles a little tighter, your breathing a little shallower, your brain a little more alert, all day, and unfortunately, all night.

For me, this felt like lying in bed with a foot on the gas pedal. Even when I wanted to sleep, my body wouldn't downshift.

It weakens your resilience to normal disruptions.

When you're fully rested, your body can absorb small disturbances without breaking stride, a late night, a stressful conversation, a shift in routine. But under chronic stress, the margin disappears. A single disruption can cause a full-night collapse, because your system has no buffer left.

This is why sleep suddenly becomes fragile.

It turns stress from a feeling into a biology.

And once that happens, the emotional, behavioral, and biological systems begin feeding each other's instability.

That's what happened to me.
One day I could bounce back.
Then suddenly I couldn't.
The signs were there long before the collapse, but I didn't know how to read them. My body was telling me it couldn't regulate itself anymore. But I kept living as though it could.

When stress reaches this depth, sleep is no longer something you "do."
It becomes something your body must relearn.
Something it must rebuild from the inside out.
Something that requires alignment across all three systems, not force, not grit, not exhaustion.

When people say they feel like they're "falling apart," they're not being dramatic. They're describing the lived experience of stress moving from the surface to the core.

The good news, what the entire Dreameaz method is built on, is that biology is not a one-way road.
What can be disrupted can be restored.
What can be learned can be unlearned.
What stress breaks, alignment can rebuild.

Chapter 6: The Emotional System

Section 1: The Racing Mind and Nighttime Rumination

There's a moment each night, somewhere between the lights going off and sleep arriving, when the body tries to hand control over to the mind. For most people, that handoff is seamless. The brain softens, thoughts drift, the edges blur, and sleep quietly takes over.

But for those living with an overloaded emotional system, that transition becomes the most volatile moment of the entire day.

For years, I didn't understand why my mind seemed to come alive the second the world went dark. I could push through the day with discipline. I could handle pressure, solve problems, make decisions, keep everything moving. But when night came, when the environment finally quieted, my mind refused to.

It didn't matter how tired I felt.
It didn't matter how early I tried to go to bed.
The moment my head hit the pillow, a new kind of alertness took over.

This is the emotional system in its purest form, unfiltered, unmasked, and uncompromising.

The Mind Accelerates When the World Slows Down

During the day, distraction does much of the heavy lifting.
You're busy. You're occupied. You're responding. You're productive. You're engaged with the world outside of you.

But at night, when the noise fades and the input stops, all the thoughts that were waiting in line suddenly rush forward.

The mind starts reviewing the day.
Then it previews the next one.
Then it replays old conversations, old mistakes, old patterns.
Then it analyzes problems you haven't solved and even ones you already did.
Then it decides to remind you of every unfinished task, every loose thread, every uncertainty.

It's like the quiet becomes a doorway, and everything you didn't have emotional space for during the day spills through it at once.

For a long time, I thought this was normal.
Just "thinking too much."
Just being "wired that way."
Just the cost of carrying heavier responsibilities.

But a racing mind at night is not personality.
It's physiology mixed with emotion.

It's the emotional system refusing to shut off because it spent the entire day in a state of heightened responsibility and never got the chance to downshift.

Rumination Isn't Worry, It's a Search for Safety

Nighttime rumination often gets mislabeled as anxiety.
And yes, sometimes it is.
But more often, it's your emotional system running a protective scan.

It's asking:

- *Did I miss something?*

- *Is everything handled?*

- *What could go wrong tomorrow?*

- *What didn't I finish?*

- *Where am I falling behind?*

- *What needs my attention?*

It feels like worry, but underneath, it's vigilance.
It's the emotional equivalent of checking the locks before going to sleep, but instead of checking your house, your mind checks everything else.

And if you've spent years being the responsible one, the fixer, the leader, the protector, the emotional system becomes conditioned to stay awake longer than it needs to. It thinks it's doing you a favor.

For me, this pattern was so familiar that I didn't even call it stress.

It was just *thinking*.

Just *processing*.

Just *how I operated*.

But rumination is the emotional system's way of saying:

"I don't feel safe enough to let go yet."

And sleep requires letting go.

Why the Mind Speeds Up Even When You're Exhausted

People often assume the racing mind is a sign of mental weakness or a lack of discipline.

It's not.

It's a sign the emotional system was carrying too much during the day and now has no place to put it.

When the lights go off and the distractions fade, your mind suddenly has the space to feel what it suppressed earlier. And because it's unfamiliar with stillness, it panics. Stillness becomes a trigger. Quiet becomes a threat.

Your emotional system interprets the dark as an invitation to sprint through every unresolved part of the day. Not to torment you, but to protect you. It believes that if it reviews everything, every risk, every scenario, every potential threat, you'll be better prepared when morning comes.

It doesn't know that what you actually need is rest.

How This Showed Up in My Own Nights

My experience was the same story millions of people live, just hidden behind a high-functioning exterior.

I'd lay down and immediately feel tension pulse through my chest. My mind would go from tired to *alert* in seconds. I'd run through everything waiting for me tomorrow, the meetings, deadlines, decisions, responsibilities, as if solving it all in my head would somehow help me sleep.

Then I'd replay things I said earlier that day.
Or things I didn't say.
Or conversations I needed to have but didn't want to.
Or scenarios that might never happen.

None of it felt optional.
The thoughts came with a kind of urgency that felt physical.

It was years before I understood the truth:

My emotional system didn't trust rest.

Rumination Isn't About the Thoughts, It's About the Load

People try to fix rumination by fighting the thoughts.
Trying to silence them.
Trying to distract from them.
Trying to out-think them.

But rumination isn't a "thought problem."
It's a *load* problem.

Your emotional system is overloaded from:

- unresolved stress

- constant responsibility

- unexpressed emotion

- daylong vigilance

- pressure you quietly carry

- patterns learned over a lifetime

When the emotional system is overloaded, it won't give the body permission to sleep because, on some level, it believes rest puts you at risk.

And until you lower that load, through emotional release, nervous system regulation, biological alignment, and behavioral stability, the mind will continue scanning when it should be settling.

The Racing Mind Isn't the Enemy, It's the Messenger

This is the part most people never hear:

Your racing mind isn't trying to sabotage your sleep.
It's trying to protect you with the only tool it knows: activity.

It's doing its best with incomplete information.

Once you realign the emotional system, once your biology and behavior begin supporting safety, routine, and predictability, the mind finally learns it doesn't have to run the night shift alone.

It finally feels safe enough to stand down.

Section 2: Anticipatory Anxiety, "What If I Don't Sleep?"

There's a unique kind of fear that only people who've struggled with sleep understand. It doesn't announce itself loudly. It doesn't rush in like panic. It slips in quietly, usually hours before bedtime, like a shadow that appears long before the sun goes down.

It's the fear behind the fear.
The worry *before* the worry.
The tension that builds not because something is wrong right now,
but because something *might* be wrong later.

It's the voice that asks:

"What if I can't sleep tonight?"

Most people never experience this.
They never think about sleep until their head hits the pillow.
They assume sleep will happen because, for most of their lives, it has.

But once sleep becomes unpredictable, even for a few nights, your emotional system learns something it was never meant to learn:

Nighttime isn't guaranteed.

For me, this shift happened quietly.
There was no dramatic moment.
Just a slow recognition that I was no longer sure what the night would bring.
Some nights I slept. Some nights I didn't. Some nights were tolerable. Others
blindsided me. And unpredictability is the perfect breeding ground for
anticipatory anxiety.

The Anxiety That Arrives Before the Night Does

Anticipatory anxiety isn't about the night itself.
It's about the *possibility* of the night going wrong.

As the evening approaches, the mind begins preparing.
Not because you want it to, but because your emotional system remembers
what happened the last time you couldn't sleep:

The frustration.
The racing thoughts.
The tossing and turning.
The adrenaline spike.
The dread of watching the clock.
The fear of how tomorrow would feel.
The exhaustion you already live too close to.

Your emotional system becomes hyper-aware of bedtime.
Not in a mindful way,
in a protective way.

A simple thought like *"I hope I sleep tonight"* slowly becomes *"What if I don't?"*
And "What if I don't?" becomes "I can't afford another bad night."
And "I can't afford another bad night" becomes "I need sleep. I need sleep."
And that need turns into pressure.
And pressure turns into tension.
And tension turns into alertness.
And alertness shuts down the very system you're trying to activate.

It's a vicious circle created by one thing:

doubt.

The moment you stop trusting your body's ability to sleep, your emotional system steps in and tries to take control, which is the one thing sleep cannot tolerate.

The Emotional System Learns the Wrong Lesson

People often think anticipatory anxiety comes from overthinking.
But it actually comes from learning.
Your emotional system remembers patterns incredibly well.

If you've had several unpredictable or difficult nights, your emotional system treats bedtime the way it would treat any unpredictable situation:

- stay alert

- stay prepared

- stay cautious

- run scenarios

- anticipate danger

- avoid surprises

It's not trying to cause distress.
It's trying to prevent it.

Your emotional system believes it is protecting you.
But this "protection" keeps your body in a mild threat state,
just activated enough to interfere with the transition into sleep.

I felt this all the time without having the words for it.
Around late afternoon, I'd feel a subtle shift inside. Not panic. Not dread.
Just a quiet tension in the background. A tightening. A mental bracing, as if my body were preparing for something.
Back then, I didn't understand it had nothing to do with my thoughts
and everything to do with conditioning.

My emotional system had learned:
nighttime equals fight.

Why You Can't Think Your Way Out of It

Most people respond to anticipatory anxiety with mental strategies:

"Don't worry about it."
"Stay calm."
"Tonight will be different."
"Just think positive."
"Don't get in your head."

But the emotional system doesn't respond to logic.
It responds to patterns.

If your emotional system expects difficulty, no amount of reassurance will override the emotional memory of previous nights. The body remembers the struggle even if the mind tries to ignore it.

You can't "think" yourself out of a state your emotional system learned through experience.

Why Anticipatory Anxiety Hits High Performers Extra Hard

Strangely, the people who struggle most with this are the people who are used to controlling everything else in their lives.

Leaders.
Athletes.
Entrepreneurs.
High achievers.
Highly responsible people.
People who've always been able to outwork, out-plan, or out-strategize difficulty.

They approach sleep the same way they approach everything:

"If it's broken, I can fix it. If it's hard, I can push through it."

But sleep is the one system in the body that rebels against force.
The more you try to control it, the more it slips away.

That's why anticipatory anxiety hits hardest for those who pride themselves on discipline.

The emotional system knows:
"Tonight is something I can't control."

And that loss of control feels threatening.

When the Fear of Not Sleeping Becomes the Reason You Can't Sleep

This is the paradox almost everyone hits:

You start fearing the nights you might not sleep.
That fear activates your emotional system.
Your emotional system triggers alertness.
Alertness blocks sleep.
The blocked sleep confirms your fear.

And so the fear grows.

You're not spiraling.
You're not dramatic.
You're not catastrophizing.

Your emotional system is trying to prevent suffering,
and accidentally causing it.

The Quiet Turning Point

The shift out of anticipatory anxiety never comes from convincing yourself
"tonight will be different."
It comes from rebuilding trust in your body,
from aligning the behavioral, biological, and emotional systems until the
emotional system no longer feels the need to interfere.

It comes from consistent routines your emotional system can rely on.
From signals of safety that sink deeper than thought.
From environments that whisper, "You don't have to stay alert anymore."
From experiences that retrain your emotional memory.

Eventually, the emotional system can unlearn its fear of the night.
It can relearn that darkness is not a threat.
That sleep is not a battle.
That the body knows what to do without intervention.

But it starts with understanding this core truth:

You're not afraid of the night.
You're afraid of what the night has done to you before.

Once we rebuild the systems underneath,
your emotional system no longer has anything to anticipate or protect you
from.

Section 3: Trauma Loops and Unresolved Stress

Not all stress comes from the present.
Some of it comes from the past, long shadows cast by old experiences that
never fully left the nervous system. Most people never realize how much their
history influences their nights, because during the day, they're too busy to feel
it. They power through. They focus. They lead. They perform. They move
fast enough that the deeper layers stay quiet.

But at night, when everything slows down, unresolved stress becomes loud.

Even if the events that shaped you are long behind you, your nervous system
may still be living as if they're active.

And that's where trauma loops begin.

Trauma Isn't Just Big Events, It's Anything Your System Never Properly Processed

When people hear the word "trauma," they think of dramatic, catastrophic
events. But the emotional system defines trauma differently. To the body,
trauma is anything that exceeded your capacity to process, regulate, or make
sense of at the time.

It can be:

- a childhood filled with unpredictability

- years of pressure or responsibility

- growing up without safety or stability

- military conditioning that rewarded vigilance

- business environments where mistakes weren't options

- relationship dynamics that eroded trust

- financial or survival stress carried for years

- losses you never slowed down long enough to feel

- conflicts you kept buried because other people counted on you

Trauma isn't about what happened.
It's about what stayed inside.

The Body Stores What the Mind Doesn't Resolve

During the day, logic runs the show.
At night, biology does.

Biology remembers.

If you grew up in an environment where you had to stay aware, stay prepared, stay ready, your nervous system learned that vigilance equals safety. Even if your adult life is stable, that old wiring remains in the background like a silent operating system.

For years, I didn't see this in myself. I thought I'd simply "moved past" the things that shaped me. I learned to work harder, to focus, to rise above, to avoid dwelling on the past.

But the nervous system doesn't move past things just because your mind says it has. It processes through the body first, and through sleep.

And when sleep becomes the one place you can no longer outrun discomfort, the old patterns appear.

Trauma Loops: When Old Wiring Shows Up in New Nights

A trauma loop isn't a conscious memory.
It's a pattern.

It feels like:

- sudden alertness for no reason

- chest tightness without a thought attached to it

- waking at the same hour every night

- a jolt of adrenaline when you're about to drift off

- feeling watched even in an empty room

- expecting something to go wrong

- lying in bed with your body braced for impact

- the mind rehearsing scenarios that don't match the moment

- restlessness that feels familiar, not situational

It's your emotional system repeating an old response because it never received a new outcome.

You don't have to be thinking about the past for the body to be reacting to it.

This was one of the hardest truths I had to accept in my own journey. I didn't feel emotionally overwhelmed. I didn't feel haunted by memories. I didn't feel fragile or upset or stuck.

What I felt was readiness.
At night, my body stayed "on" even when nothing was happening.

It took me a long time to realize this wasn't anxiety about the present,
it was the residue of years spent in environments that demanded vigilance.

Unresolved Stress Doesn't Disappear, It Accumulates

If you don't process stress in real time, the emotional system has to hold it for you. And when that holding continues for years, the brain begins looping patterns automatically.

You don't get to choose when the loop plays.
The loop chooses the moment.

And the quiet of night is the perfect moment.

Because at night:

- there are no distractions

- there is no noise

- there is no mission

- there is no task

- there is nothing external to focus on

The emotional system finally has the space to release what it carried. But if the load is too large, release becomes rumination, and rumination becomes fear, and fear becomes activation.

And activation destroys sleep.

How Trauma Loops Turn Into Sleep Patterns

Sleep is the one state where your emotional system must fully surrender. But trauma loops are built on the belief that surrender is unsafe.

So the emotional system fights the transition.

You don't feel like you're fighting anything.
You're just lying there.

But internally, your body is:

- scanning

- bracing

- stiffening

- anticipating

- replaying

- resisting the drop into vulnerability

Every time you get close to drifting off, a tiny alarm goes off. Sometimes it's a memory. Sometimes it's a physical sensation. Sometimes it's a jolt. Sometimes it's a thought that feels out of place. Sometimes it's nothing you can name.

Your emotional system is interrupting sleep because it learned that being defenseless was once dangerous.

Why High-Functioning People Are Hit Hardest

This part surprises many people:

Those who appear strongest on the outside often carry the deepest unresolved stress.

Because they never let themselves feel it.
Because they never had the space to.
Because their identity depended on pushing through.
Because people relied on them.
Because life demanded performance, not processing.

You became good at surviving through speed, focus, and control.
And those traits served you.

But when the world gets quiet, the emotional system sees its opportunity and says:

"It's finally safe to feel."

And that's when the loops appear.

The Good News: Trauma Loops Aren't Permanent

This is the part almost everyone gets wrong:

Trauma loops don't mean you're damaged.
They mean your emotional system is still trying to protect you based on old information.

When the behavioral and biological systems begin realigning,
when the emotional system receives consistent cues of safety,
when the body experiences rest without threat,
the loop begins to unwind.

It takes repetition, not force.
Ritual, not willpower.
Signals of safety, not self-criticism.

But the brain is plastic.
The emotional system is adaptable.
What was learned can be unlearned.
What was encoded can be rewritten.
What once kept you awake can eventually put you to sleep.

Section 4: Fight-or-Flight Activation After Dark

There's a version of nighttime alertness that goes far deeper than a racing mind. It's the kind of activation that doesn't feel like "thinking too much" or "being stressed." It feels physical. Instinctual. Automatic. As if some hidden switch flips on the moment the lights go off.

It's the involuntary surge, the one that feels like your body is preparing for something it can't name.

People describe it in different ways:

"I feel tired until I get into bed, then my body wakes up."
"My mind is quiet, but my chest feels active."
"I'm drifting off and suddenly I jolt awake."
"My heartbeat feels… alert."
"It's like something won't let me fall asleep."

All of these point back to a single system being activated:

your fight-or-flight circuitry.

The Body Isn't Designed to Sleep Until It Feels Safe

This is one of the most overlooked truths in all of sleep science:
Sleep is the most vulnerable thing a human being does.

When you sleep:

- your awareness drops

- your muscles release

- your senses dim

- your defenses shut down

- you lose conscious control

So the emotional system, especially the parts responsible for survival, refuses to allow sleep unless it believes the environment, the moment, and the internal state are safe.

This worked perfectly in a world filled with real dangers.
But in the modern world, the "danger" is often internal.

A racing heart.
A stressful day.
A looming deadline.
A small argument.
A spike of adrenaline.
An unresolved emotion.
A memory you didn't process.
A noise you barely registered.

All of these can trigger the same ancient circuitry your ancestors relied on to avoid being eaten in the dark.

Why It Happens More at Night

You may not notice fight-or-flight during the day.
There's too much happening.
You're moving.
You're focused.
Your attention is outward.

But at night:

- stillness highlights activation

- quiet amplifies subtle sensations

- darkness removes distractions

- your focus turns inward

- emotional residue rises to the surface

- the body realizes it can no longer outrun the day

This is why so many people say:

"I'm fine all day, but the moment I try to sleep, everything hits me."

That's not coincidence.
That's physiology.

During the day, your emotional system can postpone activation.
At night, it has nowhere else to send it.

What Fight-or-Flight Feels Like in the Body

People often think fight-or-flight is panic.
Or fear.
Or intense emotional overwhelm.

More often, it feels like:

- subtle chest tension

- elevated heart rate

- shallow breathing

- a sense of "readiness"

- difficulty exhaling fully

- warmth in the face or chest

- sudden spikes of alertness

- jolts right as you're drifting off

- restlessness that feels irrational

- tension in the solar plexus

- a sense that "something is off"

- being tired but unable to drop

It can be quiet.
It can be mild.
But mild activation is still activation.
And activation blocks sleep.

For me, this was one of the most confusing parts of the entire journey. I wasn't panicked. I wasn't having anxious thoughts. I wasn't spiraling or catastrophizing. I just felt *on*, a strange internal readiness even when my mind felt calm.

It didn't match my thoughts.
It didn't match my environment.
It didn't match my intentions.
It just lived there, beneath the surface, without explanation.

And that's because fight-or-flight doesn't begin in your thoughts.
It begins in your body.

Why High Performers Experience This the Most

If you've spent years, maybe decades, operating under pressure, responsibility, and expectation, then fight-or-flight is more than a response. It becomes a default state.

Your emotional system learns that:

- you can't afford to miss anything

- you need to stay sharp

- mistakes carry consequences

- people depend on you

- rest is a luxury

- slowing down equals falling behind

- vigilance equals safety

This conditioning doesn't disappear at bedtime.

Many high performers train their emotional systems to stay activated.
Not intentionally, just through living in environments that demand readiness.

And when the world finally gets quiet, your emotional system does what it always does:
It stays on.

Why This Creates "Sleep Starts" and Night Jolts

One of the most classic signs of nighttime fight-or-flight is the jolt, the sudden shock of wakefulness right as you begin slipping into sleep.

It feels like:

- a drop

- a spark

- a gasp

- a flinch

- a snap of awareness

- a feeling of catching yourself

It often happens because the emotional system interprets the first transition into sleep as a loss of control.

Instead of surrendering into deeper stages, the system panics, thinking:

"Wait, are we safe enough for this?"

The jolt is an interruption.
A protective reflex.
A signal that the emotional system hasn't been convinced it's time to release.

Without addressing this underlying activation, no amount of cognitive reframing will help.
The emotional system doesn't understand logic.
It understands patterns, signals, and internal cues.

The Good News: Fight-or-Flight Can Be Re-trained

This activation doesn't mean something is wrong with you.
It means your emotional system has been doing too much for too long.
It means it learned to protect you in ways that are no longer necessary.
And it means the system is primed for realignment once it receives the right signals.

The Dreameaz Method rebuilds those signals:

- predictable routines that teach the emotional system what to expect

- environmental cues that whisper safety

- breath patterns that shift you out of threat mode

- behavioral alignment that stabilizes biological rhythms

- emotional release that reduces internal load

Once those foundations are in place, nighttime activation loses its grip.

The emotional system no longer has to guard the doorway to sleep.
It finally understands that the night is not a threat.
It finally stands down.
And sleep becomes possible again, naturally, deeply, and without force.

Section 5: How Pressure Keeps the Entire System Wired

There is a specific kind of pressure that doesn't feel like panic or overwhelm. It feels like responsibility, a constant, humming awareness of everything you carry, everything expected of you, everything that cannot fall apart because too many people depend on you.

This pressure isn't dramatic.
It's not emotional in the obvious sense.
It doesn't announce itself.

It lives in the background of your life like a quiet generator, always running, always spinning, always pushing you forward. And because it blends into the pace of your days, you don't recognize it as pressure at all. You just call it *life*.

But your emotional system recognizes it.
And it responds every single day, whether you notice or not.

The Pressure to Hold Everything Together

For people who lead, build, provide, protect, or carry more weight than most, pressure becomes woven into identity.

You become the person who solves.
The person who absorbs.
The person who manages.
The person who keeps situations steady.
The person who doesn't break, because breaking isn't an option.

When that becomes your role, at work, at home, in relationships, the emotional system never truly stands down. Instead, it adapts:

- It sharpens your awareness.

- It keeps you scanning for potential problems.

- It holds tension in your muscles to keep you ready.

- It speeds up your thoughts just enough to stay ahead.

- It maintains a slight edge in your physiology so you don't miss anything.

It's trying to help.
It's trying to support the identity you've built.
It's trying to keep you functioning at the level your life demands.

But that level of activation spreads like a ripple into every other system, especially sleep.

Pressure Creates a 24/7 Readiness State

This readiness doesn't feel like stress usually does.
It doesn't come with worry or panic.
It doesn't look like emotional overwhelm.

It feels like:

- being "on" all the time

- having difficulty relaxing fully

- a buzzing under the skin

- difficulty switching tasks mentally

- feeling responsible even when nothing is happening

- not wanting to disengage because it feels unsafe

- carrying conversations, plans, and decisions in your mind even during downtime

- a belief that you have to stay ahead to keep everything stable

This state is subtle, but powerful.
It's the emotional system whispering:

"Don't slow down yet. Not now. You can rest later."

Except "later" keeps moving.
And nights become the only time left for that readiness to unwind, which is exactly why they become the hardest.

Pressure Makes Stillness Feel Dangerous

One of the strangest effects of chronic pressure is that stillness stops feeling restorative.

It feels wrong.
It feels unfamiliar.
It feels like you should be doing something.
It feels like you're dropping the ball.
It feels like you're losing momentum.
It feels like something bad might happen if you fully release.

Your emotional system interprets stillness not as rest, but as vulnerability.

So when you lie down at night, finally ready to let go, your emotional system often does the opposite. It wakes up. It sharpens. It runs diagnostics. It checks every worry, every thought, every responsibility that didn't resolve during the day.

Not because you're anxious…

…but because your emotional system fundamentally believes that *you cannot step away yet.*

How This Played Out in Your Own Life

You carried pressure through every era of your life, childhood instability, military discipline, entrepreneurship, leadership, responsibility for teams, family, clients, outcomes. You never operated in environments where letting your guard down felt like an option.

Your system learned efficiency.
It learned readiness.
It learned forward momentum.
It learned that slowing down is expensive.
It learned that rest is something you earn, not something you simply need.

So, by the time sleep began slipping away, the emotional system had built a lifetime of momentum. Nights weren't "quiet" to your body; they were the first time all day that your internal protector had a chance to speak.

And it spoke loudly.

Not through fear.
Not through panic.
But through activation, a biologically deep refusal to let you step out of the role you carried during the day.

Pressure Doesn't Just Influence Emotion, It Reshapes Biology

This is the critical link most people never learn:

Chronic emotional pressure eventually becomes physical pressure.

Over time, it reshapes:

- hormone output

- heart-rate patterns

- breathing rhythms

- muscle tension

- nervous system readiness

- inflammatory response

- temperature regulation

Which means sleep isn't just "emotionally hard" under pressure, it becomes biologically disrupted.

Your emotional system signals the biological system to stay in motion.
The biological system signals the behavioral system that rest is unsafe.
The behavioral system creates routines and habits that reinforce activation.

And suddenly, all three systems, emotional, biological, behavioral, are pulling you away from sleep at exactly the moment you need it most.

The Pattern Is Predictable, and Reversible

Once pressure builds to this level, nightly activation becomes almost automatic.
But the good news, the part most people never hear, is that this state is not permanent.

It can be unwound.

Your emotional system can learn safety again.
Your biological rhythms can stabilize.
Your behavior can send new signals.
The pressure can soften.
The readiness can fade.
The body can return to equilibrium.

This is exactly what the next chapter will show, how your deepest emotional patterns, experiences, and triggers revealed the final piece of the puzzle:

Sleep wasn't breaking because you were weak.
It was breaking because your entire system was trying to protect you.

Section 6: What Your Deepest Triggers Revealed About Sleep

There are moments in life when you think you've "handled" everything, the pressure, the responsibility, the weight you carry, until something tiny exposes the truth. A small comment. A missed email. A decision you thought wouldn't matter. A late-night thought that lingers half a second too long.
These moments feel insignificant on the surface, but they reveal the deeper patterns driving your emotional system, patterns that don't just affect your days, but shape your nights.

For years, I assumed my triggers were just products of stress or a busy life. I didn't realize they were windows into the emotional patterns that quietly hijacked my sleep.

What surprised me most was how subtle those triggers were. They didn't show up as big emotional breakdowns or dramatic panic. They arrived quietly, disguised as familiar reactions, irritability, tension, reactivity, racing thoughts, the things I told myself were "just how I'm wired."

But sleep has a way of exposing what the day hides.

The triggers you don't notice during the day are the ones that wake you at night

When you're busy, you can outrun your emotional load. But at night, when everything goes quiet, your emotional system is finally loud enough to be heard.

For me, that showed up as:

- a sudden spike of alertness right as I was drifting off

- a sharp memory or unfinished thought that pulled me wide awake

- a conversation replaying itself in loops

- a tension across my chest that I couldn't explain

- a vague sense that I "missed something" that wouldn't release

None of these felt like traditional anxiety. They felt more like a system trying to protect me from something I hadn't yet named.

What I didn't understand back then, and what most people never connect to sleep, is that triggers are not about the trigger itself. They're about what the trigger represents.

Triggers point to the stories the mind still believes

In my case, these triggers often came back to one theme:

If I don't stay alert, something will slip, and slipping is not an option.

That belief wasn't born from adult stress alone. It was shaped years earlier, through environments where awareness was survival, where missing something had consequences, where vigilance was rewarded, even necessary.

You don't consciously carry those beliefs into your adult life.
Your nervous system carries them for you.

So when a small mistake happened, or something felt out of my control, or responsibility stacked too high, I didn't just "feel stressed", I felt activated. My body hit the same internal posture it learned decades ago: *stay awake, stay sharp, stay ready.*

That posture is incompatible with sleep.

Triggers are memories of how you learned to survive

Most people think nighttime rumination is about worry or overthinking. But more often, it's your emotional system replaying the same patterns you learned a long time ago:

- anticipating

- preparing

- protecting

- scanning

- preventing

- staying ahead

Your emotional system doesn't know you're in a bed now. It only knows the rhythm your life trained it to expect.

And when you've lived a life that required strength, vigilance, and intensity, even in subtle ways, your system learns to hold those patterns long after the environment changes.

The Breakthrough: Seeing patterns instead of blaming yourself

For years, I blamed myself for these reactions. I thought:

- *Why can't I shut my mind off?*

- *Why do I replay things that don't matter?*

- *Why do small stressors hit harder at night?*

- *Why can't I just rest like everyone else?*

But when I finally stepped back and looked at the emotional system the same way I looked at the biological and behavioral ones, I saw something different:

My triggers made sense.

They weren't flaws.
They weren't weaknesses.
They weren't proof I was "wired wrong."

They were emotional habits formed over a lifetime, habits built to keep me functioning, performing, and responsible.

My emotional system wasn't trying to sabotage my sleep.
It was trying to protect me in the only way it knew how.

When you understand what your triggers are trying to do, they lose their power over your nights

This was one of the major turning points in my own recovery. Not because the triggers disappeared overnight, but because I stopped fighting them and started interpreting them.

I began seeing:

- the spike of alertness

- the sudden thought loop

- the gut-tightening memory

- the pressure in my chest

- the replayed conversation

…not as signs that something was wrong with me, but as signs that something inside me was trying to keep me safe.

And once I understood that I could work with it instead of against it.

The emotional system doesn't need to be conquered, it needs to be reassured

Most people try to "think their way" into calm.
But calm isn't created through thinking.

It's created through:

- emotional safety

- practiced transitions

- predictable rituals

- lowering internal pressure

- releasing the need to stay alert

- repairing trust in your body

- giving your system signals that night is not a threat

When your emotional system feels safe, sleep follows.
When it doesn't, sleep becomes a negotiation.

Looking back, my triggers were a map, not a failure

Every pattern I experienced pointed to one truth:
My emotional system wasn't broken. It was overloaded and untrained for rest.

This is the part most people never understand about sleep:

Your emotional triggers don't block sleep because they're powerful, they block sleep because your system hasn't learned what safety feels like at night.

And once you learn that…
everything changes.

Chapter 7: You're Not Broken, You're Misaligned

Section 1: What Sleep Actually Is

Most people think sleep is something that happens *to* you, a quiet moment when your mind shuts off and your body goes still. But that's not what sleep really is.

Sleep is not passive.
It's not "doing nothing."
It's not simply the absence of wakefulness.

Sleep is the most sophisticated, coordinated, biologically orchestrated event your body performs.

Every night, even on your worst nights, even when you swear you didn't sleep at all, your body is still fighting its way into whatever fragments of sleep it can manage.

Because here's a truth most people never hear:

Your body will always sleep, even if you don't feel it.
Even if it's broken into micro-bursts.
Even if it's incomplete.
Even if you're convinced you were awake the entire night.

You cannot "lose" the ability to sleep.
It's not a skill you forget.
It's not a function that disappears.
It's a survival mechanism as essential as breathing.

Your body would not let you live without sleep.
It cannot.
It will always find a way to rest, just not always in the way you recognize.

What happens during chronic insomnia is not the absence of sleep.
It's **the absence of deep, restorative sleep.**
It's the loss of continuity, not the loss of the system itself.

When your nervous system is misaligned, sleep becomes fragmented, shallow, inconsistent, and easily disrupted, but it does *not* disappear.

You may wake feeling like you didn't sleep.
You may have no memory of drifting.
You may only feel the exhaustion that followed.

But below your awareness, your brain was still slipping into micro-sleeps, into light stages, into brief cycles of restoration, because it had to.
Because the body cannot survive without it.

So let's remove one of the heaviest fears right here, right now:

You are not incapable of sleep.
Your biology is not refusing to sleep.
You are not staying awake for days on end.
You are sleeping, just not sleeping well.

And that changes everything.

Because if your body *still* manages to sleep while misaligned, exhausted, overwhelmed, overstimulated, and running on fragments of energy…
imagine what it can do once we realign the system.

Sleep is not a switch.
It's a symphony.

Every night, thousands of internal processes attempt to line up:

- Hormones rise and fall like tides.

- Body temperature drops in preparation for biological surrender.

- Muscles gradually release tension.

- Thoughts slow as brainwaves shift gears.

- Emotional residue from the day moves toward processing.

- Repair systems begin warming up.

Even on nights you feel like you "never slept," these systems still try.
Some succeed.
Some fail.

Some fire at the wrong time.
Some never fully activate.

When one or two systems misalign, sleep becomes inconsistent.
When several misalign, sleep becomes fragile.
When many misalign at once, sleep becomes broken into pieces, micro-cycles instead of full cycles.

But even then, it is still happening.

This is why people often say, "I swear my eyes were open all night," yet a sleep study shows they slept several hours in fragmented patterns.

Your body wasn't betraying you.
It was surviving.

Sleep is not fragile.
Sleep is quiet, and easily drowned out by louder systems such as stress, fear, hypervigilance, adrenaline, emotional load, and modern overstimulation.

And that's the key insight most people are missing:

Sleep doesn't disappear.
It gets crowded out.

Which means the path forward is not about "teaching" your body to sleep, it already knows how.
It's about **rebuilding the internal environment where sleep is allowed to do what it's designed to do.**

You aren't trying to create sleep.
You're trying to uncover it.

And once you understand that, the entire journey changes.

You stop fearing nights.
You stop panicking at 2AM.
You stop believing you're broken.
You stop thinking sleep is something you must chase or force.

You begin to see it for what it truly is:

A biological system waiting for alignment, not perfection, not performance, just alignment.

The moment you understand what sleep actually is, you reclaim the one thing insomnia takes first:
hope.

Not a fragile hope, a grounded, biological, evidence-based hope that your body still works, your systems still function, and sleep is not gone. It's simply trapped under layers of misalignment that we can unwind.

Section 2: Removing Guilt and Reframing Failure

One of the cruelest parts of losing sleep is the guilt.
People don't talk about it, but it's there, heavy, private, and corrosive.

You lie awake at night and blame yourself.

You wake up exhausted and blame yourself.

You drag through the day and blame yourself.

You hear someone say, "You just need a routine," or "You need more discipline," and suddenly your exhaustion feels like a character flaw. As if sleep were a moral achievement rather than a biological function.

And the longer the struggle lasts, the more you begin to believe the one story that does the most damage:

"This is my fault."

But it's not.
It never was.

Sleep isn't something you earn by being good enough.
It isn't a reward for discipline.
It isn't withheld because of weakness.
It doesn't improve because you beat yourself up.
And it doesn't fall apart because you failed.

Your sleep broke for reasons far bigger and far more complex than anything you did wrong.

The nervous system drifted out of alignment.
The world overloaded your circuits.
Your biology became confused.
Your emotional system stayed on guard for too long.
Your habits evolved around survival, not rest.
Your environment demanded performance at all hours.

None of that is a reflection of your character.

But guilt convinces people it is.

Guilt tells you the tension is your fault.
Guilt tells you the racing thoughts are a weakness.
Guilt tells you waking at 3AM is you "not trying hard enough."
Guilt tells you that one bad night means you're starting over.
Guilt tells you everyone else sleeps fine, so why can't you?

And guilt has a strange way of shaping identity:

"I'm a bad sleeper."
"I'm anxious."
"My mind just doesn't shut off."
"I sabotage myself."
"I must be doing something wrong."
"There's something wrong with me."

But none of that is true.

What you call "failure" is actually misalignment.
What you call "sabotage" is your biology protecting you.
What you call "weakness" is your nervous system stuck on high alert.
What you call "brokenness" is simply a system trying to operate without the conditions it needs.

You were never meant to blame yourself for a physiological process your conscious mind doesn't control.

You wouldn't blame yourself for a fever.
You wouldn't shame yourself for a strained muscle.
You wouldn't accuse yourself of "not trying hard enough" to digest food or regulate heart rate.

Yet somehow, when sleep falters, people turn on themselves.

But here's the truth that dissolves guilt the moment you let it in:

Sleep problems are not failures, they're signals.
Not judgment, information.
Not proof something is wrong with you, proof something needs attention inside you.

Your body hasn't betrayed you.
It's talking to you.

And the moment you replace guilt with understanding, everything changes.

You stop fighting yourself.
You stop fearing nights.
You stop judging your symptoms.
You stop interpreting your struggle as a personal defect.

You begin to see the real story:

Your sleep isn't broken.
Your system is misaligned.
Alignment can be restored.
And nothing about this journey requires shame.

You don't need to be punished into sleep.
You need to be supported into it.

You don't need harder routines.
You need the right ones.

You don't need perfection.
You need alignment.

You don't need to be someone else.
You need to return to the person your body still remembers how to be.

And once guilt falls away, you discover something underneath it, the thing sleep stole long before you realized:

Grace.

Grace for yourself.
Grace for your body.
Grace for the parts of you that were fighting battles you never acknowledged.

This is where transformation begins.

Section 3: The Philosophy of Realignment Over Perfection

There's a moment every exhausted person reaches, a point where the nights blend together, the days feel heavier than they should, and the simple act of trying starts to feel like its own kind of failure. I reached that point long before I had a name for it. Long before I understood what was happening inside my own body.

If you're reading this, you may have reached it too.

For most of my life, I operated under a belief that ran me straight into the ground:
If something isn't working, try harder. Push more. Tighten the grip. Control the outcome.

It's the belief that shaped my childhood.
It's the belief the military refined inside me.
It's the belief entrepreneurship reinforced.
It's the belief that carried me through every moment where falling apart wasn't an option.

And it's the belief that destroyed my sleep.

Because sleep is the one part of your life you cannot dominate through effort.

Trying harder doesn't bring it closer, it pushes it further away.
Controlling your mind doesn't calm it, it makes it louder.
Demanding your body shut down doesn't make it cooperate, it makes it brace.

I didn't know that at the time.
All I knew was that the more I fought to sleep, the worse things became.

Night after night, I'd lie in bed with this self-imposed expectation that I
needed to do everything perfectly:
perfect routine,
perfect timing,
perfect breathing,
perfect mindset,
perfect stillness.

As if perfection was the door I needed to unlock in order to get rest.

But perfection is not how sleep works.
Perfection is not how biology works.
Perfection is not how healing works.

Realignment is.

And learning that changed everything.

Realignment Isn't About Doing More, It's About Doing the Right Things in the Right Order

Realignment means understanding that your systems, behavioral, biological,
emotional, aren't broken. They're simply out of sync.

And when systems fall out of sync, the solution isn't intensity.
It's sequence.
It's pacing.
It's rhythm.

It's teaching your body how to trust the night again.

This was the part of the journey I resisted the most, because realignment
required something I'd never been taught to offer myself:

Grace.

Grace to not get it perfect.

Grace to go slow.

Grace to have off days.

Grace to recognize that biology doesn't follow motivation, it follows cues.

When your systems drift over months or years, they don't snap back because you had one good night, one good routine, or one motivated moment. They shift gradually, steadily, predictably, the same way they drifted in the first place.

Realignment is a process, not an event.

Perfection Demands Control, Realignment Restores Ease

Perfection says:

- "Don't mess up your routine."

- "Don't drink that coffee."

- "Don't stay up too late."

- "Don't think too much."

- "Don't break your streak."

- "Don't let your mind wander."

Perfection turns sleep into a test.

Realignment says:

- "Let's create a rhythm your body recognizes."

- "Let's build cues your system trusts."

- "Let's repair what overwork broke."

- "Let's soften the nights instead of forcing them."

- "Let's make your biology feel safe again."

- "Let's bring your systems back into harmony."

Realignment turns sleep into a natural response again.

For the first time in my life, I stopped chasing sleep like a goal and started building the conditions for sleep to return on its own.

This isn't just a philosophical shift, it's a biological one.
Because when you stop demanding perfection, your nervous system stops bracing for failure.

When you stop chasing sleep, your mind stops fearing the night.

When you stop performing for rest, your body stops resisting it.

Realignment Is the First Doorway to Hope

When I finally understood that my systems needed alignment, not discipline…
that my body needed guidance, not force…
that my exhaustion wasn't a verdict, but a signal…

I felt something I hadn't felt in years:

Hope.
Not vague hope.
Not "maybe one day" hope.
Not "if I get lucky" hope.

But grounded, biological hope, the kind you feel when you finally understand the mechanics beneath your suffering.

Because once you understand that your sleep loss isn't a mystery…
isn't a punishment…
isn't an identity…
isn't proof of weakness…

…it becomes solvable.

Sleep isn't magic.
It isn't luck.

It isn't something you earn by being perfect.
It isn't something you lose because you "couldn't handle life."

It's a system.

A system you can rebuild.

A system that wants to heal.

A system that already knows the way back.

Realignment isn't about becoming a different person.

It's about becoming the version of yourself your biology was always designed to support.

And once you learn that, once you feel it, the night stops being a threat.

It becomes a home you're learning to return to.

Section 4: The Hope You Didn't Know You Still Had

Hope is a strange thing when you've been exhausted for a long time.
It shrinks without you noticing.
It fades in small, almost polite increments, the same way sleep does.

You don't wake up one day and decide to give up.
You simply stop expecting things to get better.

You stop believing tomorrow will feel different.
You stop believing your body will ever calm down.
You stop believing your mind will ever go quiet.
You stop believing sleep will ever feel natural again.

And maybe most painfully, you stop believing *you* can be fixed.

Not because you're dramatic.
Not because you're negative.
But because night after night, your body is giving you evidence that it no longer remembers how to rest.
Or so it seems.

This section exists to correct that lie.

Because what you think is the end of sleep…
is often the beginning of understanding.

The Hope Hidden Inside Your Biology

Most people don't realize something simple but incredibly important:

Your body is sleeping more than you think.

Even when you feel awake.
Even when it feels fragmented.
Even when your mind is racing.
Even when you swear you got "zero sleep."

The body cannot survive without sleep.
It will take micro-sleeps… momentary dips… fragmented cycles… anything it can get.

It's not the kind of sleep you want.
It's not the kind that restores you.
But it proves something critical:

Your sleep machinery is still alive.
It's still firing.
It's still trying.
It has not given up on you, not for a moment.

And that means you're not starting from zero.
You're starting from misalignment.

That is a profoundly hopeful place to begin.

Your Systems Aren't Broken, They're Waiting

Long before I understood realignment, I spent too many nights believing something inside me had snapped permanently.
Every failed attempt felt like proof.
Every morning I woke up exhausted felt final.
Every night that ended in frustration felt like another step away from ever being "normal" again.

But biology doesn't work like that.

The Three Systems, behavioral, biological, emotional, never actually break.
They scatter.
They drift.
They fall out of sync like instruments in an orchestra that can no longer hear one another.

The music disappears,
but the instruments remain intact.

When you learn how to bring those instruments back into harmony, when you create the right cues, the right timing, the right rhythm, the music returns.

Not all at once.
Not perfectly.
But unmistakably.

That's what this book is walking you toward:
the exact point where your systems begin speaking to each other again.

Hope Doesn't Come From Trying Harder, It Comes From Understanding

For years, I tried to force myself to sleep.
Force never works.
Force creates fear.
Fear creates pressure.
Pressure activates the nervous system.
And activation blocks sleep.

That loop steals hope from millions of people:

- They try harder.

- They sleep worse.

- They blame themselves.

- They try even harder.

- It collapses again.

The moment you understand that your systems simply need realignment, not perfection, something inside you loosens.
A door opens.
Your body feels less hunted.
Your mind stops bracing.

Hope doesn't come from wishing.
It comes from clarity.

Clarity gives you direction.
Direction gives you confidence.
Confidence gives you calm.
Calm gives you the first real foothold back into sleep.

The Night Is Not the Enemy Anymore

When you've suffered long enough, nighttime becomes a threat.
You dread it.
You feel it approach.
Your mind tightens as the sun goes down.

But that changes the moment you realize something profound:

Your body remembers.
It knows how to fall asleep.
It knows how to stay asleep.
It knows how to repair itself.

It knows how to shut down.
It knows how to return to equilibrium.

It has simply forgotten the sequence.

This book teaches you the sequence.
This method restores it.
And once the sequence comes back online, sleep returns as naturally as breathing, because sleep is not something you chase.
It is something that emerges when systems fall back into harmony.

The Hope You Didn't Know You Still Had

The hope is this:

You are not fighting a broken body.
You are rebuilding a misaligned one.

You are not starting at rock bottom.
You are starting from a system that has been trying to protect you for years.

You are not failing.
You are adapting.
Now you're learning to adapt in a new direction.

The night is not a battlefield.
It's an environment your body is relearning how to trust.

And the moment that trust starts to return, even in the smallest ways, you begin to feel something you may not have felt in a very long time:

Relief.
Safety.
Lightness.
Rest. Real rest.

When you feel it for the first time, even once, hope stops being theoretical.
It becomes real.

And real hope makes sleep possible again.

Chapter 8: Identify Your Sleep Breakers

Section 1: The Dreameaz Sleep Breakers Model™, The Lens That Changes Everything

Most people who struggle with sleep can describe their nights in vivid detail, the tossing, the racing mind, the early waking, the frustration, but they can't describe the underlying mechanism. They feel lost inside their own experience, unable to name what's happening or why.

And you can't fix what you can't name.

That's where everything begins to shift.

The Dreameaz Sleep Breakers Model™ exists because for decades the world has taught people to focus on **symptoms**, not systems.
You lie awake at night and think the problem is the awareness of being awake.
You wake at 3AM and think the problem is the moment you opened your eyes.
You collapse into bed exhausted and think the problem is your willpower.

But none of those are the problem.
They are the messages.
They're the smoke, not the fire.

Underneath every sleep struggle sits a root cause, a structural disruption in one of your three sleep systems:

- **Behavioral System**

- **Biological System**

- **Emotional System**

But here's the part almost no one ever tells you:

Most people have no idea which system is actually breaking their sleep.

They treat biological problems as emotional ones.
They treat emotional overload as behavioral failure.
They treat behavioral patterns as personal flaws.

They treat apnea as insomnia.
They treat hyperarousal as bad habits.

They throw solutions at the wrong root, get nowhere, and assume the issue is them.

It never was.

The Dreameaz Sleep Breakers Model™ puts an end to that confusion by giving you something you've never had before:

A map of your sleep struggle, clear, organized, specific, and fixable.

Why "Sleep Breakers" Matter

Think of sleep like a bridge connecting your daytime and nighttime states.
Most people try to reinforce the bridge itself.
They change pillows.
Adjust routines.
Try supplements.
Download apps.
Buy trackers.

But the bridge isn't the problem.
It's the pressure underneath it, the weight on the foundation, that makes it unstable.

Sleep Breakers are the unseen forces pulling your sleep off balance:

- The thoughts that spike your alertness right as you're trying to drift off.

- The cortisol surge at 2 or 3AM.

- The airway that collapses without warning.

- The subtle behaviors that send the wrong cues.

- The emotions your nervous system doesn't know how to put down.

- The physical stress your body hasn't discharged in years.

Most people focus on bedtime.
Sleep Breakers often begin at **10AM, 2PM, 5PM, after dinner**, or even **before you've left bed that morning**.

The magic of the Sleep Breakers Model is this:

It shows you what's breaking your sleep before you even get to the night.

Once you see it, you can't unsee it, and you'll never think about sleep the same way again.

How the Model Works

Every sleep struggle falls into one or more of these core categories:

1. Falling Asleep Breakers
These are the forces that make your mind feel "too awake," your body too tense, or your system too activated to transition.

2. Night Awakening Breakers
These are the disruptions that force you out of sleep cycles, from cortisol spikes to blood sugar crashes to emotional surges.

3. Early Waking Breakers
These occur when your circadian rhythm fires the "wake" signal too early or your nervous system refuses to re-enter sleep.

4. Mind Spiraling Breakers
These happen when your brain enters loop-mode, analyzing, replaying, predicting, and won't release control.

Each category corresponds to a specific type of dysfunction in your Three Systems:
Behavioral → Biological → Emotional.

This is where people finally start to feel relief, because they can see their nights as patterns, not mysteries.

Why This Model Is the Turning Point of the Book

Until now, you've been learning *why* your systems collapse.
You've been learning the science, the story, the emotional weight of sleeplessness.
You've walked through your own history and recognized how the pieces fell apart.

But Chapter 10 is where you finally take control.

This model gives you:

- **language** for what's happening,

- **structure** for diagnosing it,

- **precision** for identifying your root cause,

- **clarity** for what to fix first,

- **and relief** knowing there is a path.

Not vague.
Not one-size-fits-all.
Not theoretical.

But your sleep, your system, your story.

The Promise of the Dreameaz Sleep Breakers Model™

The promise of this model is simple:

Once you identify your Sleep Breakers, you can dismantle them, one by one, until sleep becomes natural again.

Not forced.
Not medicated.
Not chased.

Natural.

This chapter is where the healing begins.

Section 2: Falling Asleep Breakers, The First Fracture Point

For most people, the sleep struggle doesn't begin at 3 AM.
It begins in the very first moments of the night, the transition from doing to being, from motion to stillness, from the external world to the internal one.

That transition is where the first fracture usually appears.
It's where your systems either fall into alignment… or begin to drift.

For years, I didn't understand this.
I thought my problem was the middle of the night, the jolting wake-ups, the spirals, the racing thoughts. But long before those patterns took root, something else was already breaking down:

I had lost the ability to fall asleep cleanly.

Not dramatically.
Not all at once.
Not in a way I even recognized as a problem.

It began with a feeling I brushed off a hundred times:
Why does my mind feel louder at night?
Why does my body feel restless when I'm this tired?
Why does it take me longer to shut down than it used to?

At the time, I chalked it up to stress.
Or responsibility.
Or the grind of building businesses, raising a family, carrying weight that never felt fully put down.

But falling asleep is actually a very delicate shift, a biological handoff from wakefulness to rest, and when your systems aren't aligned, that handoff starts failing in subtle ways long before the rest of your sleep collapses.

This is the point most people miss.
This is the first real break in the chain.

And if you don't identify what's disrupting this transition, everything after that becomes harder, noisier, more fragile, and more unpredictable.

The Real Reason Falling Asleep Becomes Difficult

Falling asleep isn't about exhaustion.
It's not even about quieting thoughts.
It's a physiological transition, a downshifting of the body's entire operating system.

For the shift to happen smoothly, three things must occur:

1. **Your behavioral cues have to signal "the day is done."**

2. **Your biological rhythms have to line up behind that signal.**

3. **Your emotional system has to release its grip on control.**

When even one of those systems refuses the handoff, your ability to fall asleep becomes disrupted.
When all three resist?
Falling asleep becomes a nightly battlefield.

Most people think the problem is the thoughts.
But thoughts are almost never the root.
They're the alarm bell.
They're the symptom of systems firing at the wrong time.

Falling Asleep Breakers show you what's going wrong *behind* the thoughts.

The Four Core Falling Asleep Breakers

Every person who struggles with falling asleep has one or more of these forces working against them.
And the moment you learn to recognize them, everything starts making sense.

1. The Wired Body (Biological System)

This is when your body is tired but your physiology is still in "go-mode", heart rate elevated, cortisol drifting too high, temperature not dropping, muscles tensely holding the day.

You're trying to sleep in a body that believes it needs to stay operational.

I lived like this for years without realizing it. My body didn't trust the night because every day felt like a mission that never ended. My internal alerts were still firing long after I turned the lights out.

2. The Spinning Mind (Emotional System)

This is the classic loop:

- replaying the day

- predicting tomorrow

- worrying about sleep

- analyzing sensations

- negotiating with yourself

It's not overthinking.
It's your emotional system refusing to release control.
You don't have a "thinking problem."
You have a hyperactivated survival system.

3. The Wrong Cues (Behavioral System)

This is when your behaviors unintentionally tell your brain to stay awake:

- bright light

- late screens

- erratic routines

- eating too late

- working too close to bedtime

- lying in bed awake for long stretches

These patterns confuse your biological rhythm and delay the sleep switch.

4. The Hidden Fears (Emotional + Biological)

This one is the most misunderstood.

Sometimes falling asleep becomes difficult because the body doesn't feel safe letting go.

Not unsafe in a dramatic way, unsafe in a subtle, physiological way:

- fear of not sleeping

- fear of losing control

- fear of the night

- fear of what waking up exhausted means for tomorrow

- fear rooted in old memories or old environments

For me, this one ran deep, all the way back to childhood nights spent quietly bracing for sounds, arguments, unpredictability. My body learned early that nighttime required vigilance.

Years later, that vigilance disguised itself as "stress" or "busy thoughts," but underneath it was the same instinct:
don't fully let go.

Why This Breaker Matters So Much

Because falling asleep is the first domino.

If this transition is compromised:

- your nervous system never fully drops

- your cortisol drifts too high

- your REM becomes delayed

- your deep sleep becomes shallow

- your night wakings become more frequent

- your early mornings become earlier

- your entire next day becomes unstable

- and your confidence in your body dissolves

You begin thinking you have insomnia.
You begin thinking your mind is broken.
You begin thinking sleep is slipping away.

But really, it's just one misaligned transition, the first transition, sending shockwaves through everything else.

The good news?

Once you identify your Falling Asleep Breakers, you can repair that transition. And when the first handoff becomes smooth, the rest of the night has a fighting chance to follow.

This is where real improvement begins.

Section 3: Night Awakening Breakers, The Disruptions That Shatter the Night

If falling asleep is the first fracture point, nighttime awakenings are the fractures that hurt the most.

There's something uniquely disorienting about waking up in the middle of the night.
It hits a deeper part of you, the part that was finally off-duty, finally surrendered, finally quiet.

Then suddenly…
you're awake.
Alert.
Confused.
Heart beating too fast.
Mind trying to make sense of the moment.
Body pulled out of rest like it stepped on a landmine.

For millions of people, **this** is the moment where sleep feels most fragile, and where the fear of the night begins to form.

I lived that cycle far longer than I ever admitted.
Not every night, but enough nights.
The kind of nights where your eyes snap open and you feel instantly behind, behind on rest, behind on recovery, behind on the demands of tomorrow.

It's like waking up mid-fall.
Nothing dangerous is happening, but your body reacts like there is.

Night awakenings aren't random.
They aren't "just stress."
They aren't a personality trait.
And they aren't failure.

They are signals, precise ones, pointing directly to the system that's misaligned.

Most people never decode them.
After tonight, you will.

What Night Wakings Actually Are

Waking up in the night is your body sending up a flare.

Not because it wants to punish you.
But because your systems, behavioral, biological, emotional, hit a point where they could no longer maintain balance.

Every night waking has a cause.
Every cause has a pattern.
Every pattern maps back to a specific Sleep Breaker.

Once you understand the language your body is speaking, these awakenings stop feeling terrifying and start feeling diagnostic.

The Four Core Night Awakening Breakers

1. The Cortisol Spike, "Jolt Awake" Nights

This is the classic 1–3 AM wakeup.

You're asleep.
Then suddenly you're up, wired, alert, and confused how you went from calm to wide awake in seconds.

This is not psychological.
It's hormonal.

When cortisol rises at the wrong time, you're yanked out of sleep as if someone pulled an internal alarm.

Why it happens:

- chronic stress

- late-night work

- emotional overload

- inconsistent sleep timing

- late meals or alcohol

- unresolved fear-based states carried from childhood

- a circadian rhythm stuck in "nighttime vigilance mode"

This was one of my biggest patterns during my burnout years.
Not fear, *activation*.
My body was still running missions long after I went to bed.

2. The Blood Sugar Drop, "Adrenaline Wake-Up" Nights

This one is sneaky.

You don't feel hungry.
You don't feel panicked.
You just wake up suddenly, often with:

- a pounding heart

- heat in the chest

- slight sweating

- a feeling that something is off

It's not anxiety.
It's biochemistry.

A blood sugar dip causes adrenaline to surge to stabilize you, and that surge wakes you up.

Why it happens:

- eating too little

- eating too late

- eating high-sugar meals

- alcohol

- intense stress days

- disrupted metabolism

It often masquerades as "middle-of-the-night anxiety," when really it's physiology trying to keep you alive.

3. The Hyperactivated Mind, "Brain Turns On" Nights

You wake up slowly…
but once you're awake, your mind starts spinning almost instantly.

Planning.
Analyzing.
Replaying.
Solving tomorrow's problems at 2 AM like they're due in an hour.

This is not mental weakness.
It's emotional circuitry firing at the wrong time.

Why it happens:

- unresolved worry loops

- anticipatory anxiety

- nighttime hypervigilance

- perfectionism

- chronic responsibility

- childhood conditioning where nighttime was unsafe

- the identity of "I must stay ahead"

I lived this one on and off for decades without realizing it.
It wasn't anxiety, it was old vigilance being activated in a new life.

4. The Oxygen Disruption, "Micro-Awakening" Nights

This is the most overlooked, and for many, the most life-changing once discovered.

These awakenings don't feel dramatic.
They feel like:

- shallow sleep

- waking multiple times without knowing why

- waking unrefreshed

- waking with a dry mouth

- waking with chest tightness

- waking with a headache

- waking groggy even after long hours in bed

This is often the result of airway collapse or reduced oxygen, even mild cases.

It doesn't always look like full sleep apnea.
Sometimes it's just enough airway restriction to repeatedly pull you out of deeper sleep cycles.

This was a major part of my own story, one I ignored for far too long because I assumed my nights were "stress-based."
It wasn't until I addressed the underlying breathing issue that a whole category of night awakenings finally stopped sabotaging me.

Why Night Wakings Feel So Personal

No moment in the sleep struggle attacks your confidence like waking up in the middle of the night.

It makes you question everything:

- your resilience

- your discipline

- your biology

- your sanity

- your entire relationship with rest

This is the moment people start fearing sleep.
This is the moment the night becomes something to endure instead of something to trust.
This is the moment routines get thrown out, frustration builds, and doubt spreads.

But here's the pivot,

Night awakenings aren't proof of failure. They're proof of signals.

Signals that can be interpreted.
Signals that can be resolved.
Signals that point directly to the system that needs realignment.

Night wakings are not the enemy.
They are the map.

The Most Important Line in This Section

You are not waking up because you can't sleep.
You are waking up because something in your body is trying to communicate.

Once you understand the language, you stop fearing the night.
You start listening to it.
You start responding to it.
You start correcting the root cause.

That's where healing begins.

Section 4: Early Waking Breakers, When the Morning Comes Too Soon

There's a particular kind of exhaustion that comes from waking up too early, not the kind where your alarm surprises you, but the kind where your eyes open hours before you intended, and you know instantly:

"This isn't enough. I'm not done."

Early waking has a different emotional weight than trouble falling asleep or middle-of-the-night awakenings.
Those disruptions feel frustrating.
This one feels defeating.

It feels like the night betrayed you.
Like your body gave up halfway through the job.
Like rest slipped through your fingers even though you were finally sleeping.

I went through stretches where this early waking felt relentless, waking at 4:30AM with no reason, waking with tension in my chest, waking with a sense of unfinished rest that no amount of willpower could push back down.

At first, it feels like a glitch.
Then it starts feeling like a pattern.
Eventually, it can start feeling like a limitation, something built into you.

And that's exactly what makes early waking so psychologically damaging. It convinces you that sleep is something you can't hold onto.

But early waking is not random.
It is one of the most predictable patterns in the entire landscape of sleep disruption, and one of the easiest to interpret once you understand the systems behind it.

What Early Waking Actually Means

Early waking happens when your body switches into "wake mode" before your sleep cycles are complete.

Why?
Because something in your system is firing too early, or something that *should* fire isn't firing at all.

This is not laziness.
Not aging.
Not a "morning person" identity.
Not stress alone.
It's a system firing out of sequence.

Once you identify which system is misfiring, you can correct it, often shockingly fast.

The Three Core Early Waking Breakers

1. The Circadian Jump-Start, Your Internal Clock Is Running Ahead

This is the most common cause of early waking.

Your circadian rhythm, the timing system that governs sleep, energy, digestion, hormones, and temperature, starts its "wake-up" sequence too early.

You're not waking early because you're rested.
You're waking early because your biological clock thinks it's time.

Signs this is your breaker:

- You wake around the same time every morning, even on weekends

- The waking feels abrupt, not groggy

- You feel alert at first, then exhausted later

- You fall asleep easily at night but can't sustain the sleep window

Why it happens:

- late-night screens

- inconsistent sleep schedules

- too much light exposure at night

- not enough morning light

- cortisol rhythms shifting forward

- chronic stress pushing your "wake signal" earlier

This was one of the earliest signs in my own downfall, waking like a machine at a time I didn't choose, as if my body was on a schedule I no longer recognized.

2. The Activated Nervous System, The Body Tries to End the Night Early

Think of early waking like a nervous system "bailout", a premature escape from deeper sleep because your body doesn't feel fully safe staying there.

This doesn't mean danger.
It means **activation**.

Signs:

- You wake with tension

- Your breathing feels shallow

- You feel "ahead of yourself" mentally

- Thoughts turn on quickly

- You can't drop back down once you're up

This happens when:

- you've carried stress for too many days in a row

- you fall asleep in a sympathetic state (wired, rushed, tense)

- your system fears losing control

- unresolved emotional weight rises closer to morning

It's the nervous system saying:
"We've slept enough to survive, let's get moving."
even though you haven't.

3. The Recovery Failure, Your Sleep Didn't Go Deep Enough to Sustain Itself

This is the sleeper who sleeps 7 or 8 hours but wakes feeling un-rested… every single time.

It's also the person who wakes at 4 or 5AM because their sleep cycles never stabilized.

This happens when:

- breathing disruptions fragment sleep

- you never reach deep, slow-wave sleep

- REM is disrupted

- inflammation or stress blocks deeper cycles

- the body "aborts mission" because the quality wasn't there

People often blame themselves for this type of waking:

- "I must be getting older."

- "My sleep is just changing."

- "This is who I am now."

It's not who you are.
It's a biological pattern.
And biological patterns can be corrected.

Why Early Waking Hurts Your Confidence the Most

When you can't fall asleep, you tell yourself you'll try harder tomorrow.
When you wake in the middle of the night, you think you can fight your way back down.

But early waking leaves you with nothing to negotiate.
The night is over, even if your body isn't ready.

This is where people start telling themselves dangerous stories:

- "My body doesn't know how to sleep anymore."

- "I'm losing the ability to rest."

- "I'm waking earlier every year, maybe this is my new normal."

No.
It's not your new normal.
It's your current pattern.

And patterns change the moment the system behind them shifts.

The Most Important Truth About Early Waking

You're not waking early because your sleep is broken.
You're waking early because your **systems aren't synchronized.**

When your circadian rhythm, nervous system, and sleep architecture fall back into alignment, the early wake-ups stop.

Not gradually.
Often quickly.

Your body wants to stay asleep.

It simply needs the right timing, the right cues, and the right conditions to trust the later hours of the night again.

Section 5: Mind Spiraling Breakers, When Thoughts Become the Second Night

If falling asleep is the first battle
and staying asleep is the second,
mind spiraling is the third,
the enemy that doesn't show up in your body first,
but in your thoughts.

This is the part of the night where it feels like your mind hijacks the wheel, turns the lights on inside your skull, and decides to run back every conversation, every mistake, every possibility, every task, and every fear in the quietest hours of your life.

And the worst part?

You often can't tell whether your thoughts are waking you
or whether waking up is giving your thoughts the chance to take over.

Mind spiraling is one of the most misunderstood sleep disruptors because it *feels* mental, as if your brain simply refuses to "behave."

But spiraling is not a thinking problem.
It's a **system problem**
that shows up through thoughts.

I lived through years of this without even realizing it was part of my sleep pathology.
To me, it just felt like my identity,
like I was the kind of person who needed to think through everything,
who needed to prepare,
who couldn't shut down because shutting down felt too risky.

Only later did I understand:
it wasn't personality.
It was physiology.
It was emotional patterning.
It was misalignment.

Mind spiraling is the final and most painful Sleep Breaker because it doesn't just steal sleep, it steals peace.

What Mind Spiraling Really Is

Mind spiraling happens when your emotional system remains active while the rest of your body tries to downshift.

Which means:

- your thoughts aren't the cause of the problem

- they are the *output* of an activated emotional system

The more you try to stop spiraling,
the faster the spiraling becomes.

Because the moment you try to control your thoughts,
your emotional system receives the message:
"We are not safe."

And once safety is questioned, even subtly,
the mind does what it was designed to do:
protect, anticipate, analyze, prepare.

This is not dysfunction.
This is survival software.
It's just running at the wrong time.

The Four Core Mind Spiraling Breakers

1. The Anticipatory Loop, "What If I Don't Sleep?"

This is by far the most common.

It starts innocently:
"I hope I can sleep tonight."

Then it shifts:
"I really need sleep tonight."

Then:
"If I don't sleep tonight, tomorrow's ruined."

And eventually:
"What if I never sleep normally again?"

That thought,
that specific thought,
has kept more people awake than caffeine, screens, stress, and noise
combined.

Anticipatory looping makes the brain believe the night is a test.
And the minute the night becomes a test,
sleep becomes impossible.

2. The Responsibility Spiral, "Everything Depends on Me"

This one hits high performers, leaders, parents, and protectors.

Your mind uses the silence of the night to:

- solve tomorrow

- plan contingencies

- analyze every angle

- rehearse conversations

- anticipate problems before they happen

It feels productive.
It feels necessary.
It feels like you're staying ahead.

But it's actually your emotional system refusing to release control.

3. The Trauma-Echo Spiral, Old Stress in New Nights

This one is subtle but powerful.

Your mind isn't replaying the past directly.
It's replaying the *patterns* of the past:

- hypervigilance

- readiness

- scanning

- bracing

- expecting disruption

You don't think you're reliving anything.
But your emotional system is running an old program:
"Nighttime requires caution."

This is especially common in people who grew up in instability or unpredictability, like you did.

4. The Sensation Spiral, "Why Does My Body Feel Like This?"

This is the spiral that begins in the body and moves into the mind:

- a flutter in the chest

- a warm rush

- a muscle twitch

- a shift in breathing

- a flicker of adrenaline

If you're already sensitized by sleep struggles, these neutral sensations can trigger spiraling:

"Is this happening again?"
"Am I waking up?"
"Why do I feel this?"
"Is something wrong?"
"Can I stop this?"

Your attention becomes a magnifying glass.
The more you focus on a sensation, the more intense it becomes.
The more intense it becomes, the more you spiral.
The more you spiral, the more awake you become.

Why Mind Spiraling Feels So Personal

Unlike other sleep disruptions, spiraling feels like it comes from inside you, like it reveals something flawed or defective about your mind.

People say things like:

- "My brain hates me."

- "Why can't I control my thoughts?"

- "What's wrong with me?"

- "Why am I wired like this?"

- "Why can't I switch off like other people?"

But mind spiraling is not a personality problem.
It is not a flaw.
It is not a lack of willpower.
And it's not a sign of "losing it."

Mind spiraling is nothing more than emotional misalignment leaking into the night.

Your brain is not working against you.
It's working *for you,*

just in the wrong sequence,
at the wrong time,
under the wrong conditions.

The Most Important Truth About Mind Spiraling

You are not spiraling because you're broken.
You are spiraling because your emotional system is still "on,"
even when the rest of your systems are trying to turn "off."

Once your systems realign,
once safety is restored,
once cues are consistent,
once biology and behavior fall into rhythm again,

your mind doesn't have to "be quiet."
It becomes quiet on its own.

Thoughts stop spiraling when your systems stop fighting each other.

That's the breakthrough.

And now that you've identified all four categories of Sleep Breakers,
falling asleep,
night awakenings,
early waking,
and spiraling,

Chapter 9: Realigning the Systems

There comes a point in every sleep struggle where you stop feeling tired and start feeling defeated. Not because your body is weak, but because your systems have been pulled out of rhythm for so long that you no longer remember what a normal night feels like.

But here's the truth no one tells you:
Your body hasn't forgotten how to sleep.
It's just been surviving.

What you're about to do is guide it back.

Sleep returns when the systems that support it, your Behavioral, Biological, and Emotional Systems, begin working together again. And while all three matter, the Behavioral System is the first one to fall apart and the first one to repair. It's the system your body listens to most directly, because it lives in your actions, your pace, your patterns, and the small rituals you repeat without thinking.

Rebalancing this system isn't about willpower or strict rules. It's about giving your body the rhythm it has been missing, the rhythm that once told your brain, *"The day is ending. You're safe now."*
And when your brain hears that message again, sleep begins to return in ways that surprise you.

Section 1: Rebalancing the Behavioral System

If you're like most people who struggle with sleep, you've spent months, maybe years, blaming your mind or your body. You've wondered what's wrong with you. You've replayed every bad night and every failed attempt to "just relax." You've tried harder than anyone around you realizes.

But sleep isn't something you can force.
It's something your body allows when the environment feels safe.

And over time, your Behavioral System, the patterns you've lived in, has been teaching your body the opposite message:

Stay alert. Stay ready. Don't release.

Not because you chose those patterns.
Because life demanded them.

You pushed through late work.
You handled crises at all hours.
You used your bed as the only quiet place to think.
You scrolled to numb the noise in your mind.
You carried stress into the night because there was nowhere else to put it.
You adapted in the only way you could.

Your Behavioral System learned from it all.

Now your nights reflect the story your days have been telling.

The good news is that patterns can be rewritten.
Your Behavioral System can be recalibrated.
And when it is, your body begins to let go again.

This is how you rebuild the story your body listens to.

The Momentum of the Day

Sleep doesn't begin at night.
It begins in the morning, with the momentum you create.

In the worst periods of my own insomnia, mornings were the hardest. I'd wake up exhausted, angry at the night I just lived through, convinced the day was already lost because I felt hollow. Those mornings taught my body inconsistency; they set the wrong tone. If I woke at 6 a.m. one day and 10 a.m. the next, my internal clock never knew what to expect. The nights reflected that confusion.

What your body wants most is predictability.
What your sleep wants most is timing.
And you create both the moment you open your eyes.

That's why the Day Anchor is so powerful. It doesn't just start your day, it repairs the foundation your sleep rests on.

The Day Anchor

Rebuilding your body's sense of time.

Think of the Day Anchor as the first domino. You push it, and a cascade of internal signals begins to reorder themselves.

When you wake up around the same time each morning, your body starts learning the rhythm it forgot. If you step into light early, that light hits the part of your brain that sets your biological clock. If you move, even lightly, your nervous system interprets it as a sign of stability.

This anchor is not about perfection.
It's about consistency.

Wake up at a time your life can support. Don't punish yourself for bad nights. Wake up anyway. Open a window. Step outside for a moment. Stretch. Breathe. Drink water. Eat something small.

Each of these actions says to your body:
"The day begins now. You can stop drifting."

People underestimate this step because it seems too simple. But when your mornings stabilize, melatonin begins releasing closer to where it should. Energy rises when it's meant to. Sleep pressure, the natural tiredness that builds throughout the day, starts increasing steadily again.

This is how your nights begin to shift before the sun even sets.

The Evening Anchor

The descent from intensity to grounding.

Evenings used to be my danger zone. I didn't understand what I was doing wrong, why my mind exploded with tension the moment the house got quiet. I didn't want to admit it, but I was carrying the entire day into the night without transition.

Your nervous system can't go from full speed to stillness without a bridge. You need a descent, not a drop-off.

This is what the Evening Anchor creates.

It's the period where you teach your brain that the day is ending. Not through meditation or forced relaxation, but through the tone of your environment:

- Lights dimming

- Volume lowering

- Your pace slowing

- Tension releasing from your shoulders

- Tasks being closed instead of carried

- Small rituals signaling completion

At first, this can feel unnatural, especially if you've lived in chronic stress. You might feel restless or impatient. That's normal. It's simply your body adjusting to a slower rhythm it hasn't experienced in a long time.

But with each evening, your internal gears learn to shift earlier.
Your adrenaline begins to drop sooner.
Your mind becomes less reactive.
Your body softens into the night instead of resisting it.

This anchor is how you reclaim the transition modern life took away from you.

The Night Anchor

The conditioned script that leads you into rest.

Your brain learns through repetition. It waits for patterns. It thrives on cues. And the Night Anchor is the most powerful signal you can give it, because it creates a predictable path toward shutdown.

The Night Anchor is a simple sequence you perform in the same order every night. It can be three steps or five, as long as it is consistent.

Think of it like a movie your brain has seen a hundred times. With each scene, it knows what comes next. With each cue, it begins preparing for the ending.

A warm shower, then dim lights.
Brush your teeth, then read something calming.
Slow stretching, then the same blanket, the same lamp, the same environment.

This ritual becomes a form of behavioral conditioning.
Your brain associates these steps with "sleep is coming."
Your nervous system hears the same message every night.

And slowly, your body begins responding before you reach the final step.

Rebuilding the Bed Association

Teaching your brain that your bed no longer equals battle.

If you've struggled with sleep, you know the feeling, the dread that settles in when you walk into your bedroom, the pressure of "I have to sleep," the tension that rises the moment you lie down. This is learned association, not personal failure.

Your brain has paired your bed with wakefulness.

You've rehearsed stress, fear, worry, frustration, problem-solving, and waiting in that space. Your body learned that the bed is a place where the mind activates.

To rebuild this association, you must stop rehearsing the old story.

If you lie down and your mind ramps up, don't stay there fighting it. Fighting only deepens the association. Instead, get up gently. Sit somewhere dim. Read a page or two of something neutral. Let your nervous system settle. Then return.

What you're doing is breaking a pairing your brain has held onto for years.

And when that pairing dissolves, your bed becomes safe again.
Safe beds invite sleep.
Unsafe beds invite vigilance.

This is one of the most transformative shifts in the entire model.

The Internal Shift

You'll begin noticing small changes before the big ones.

Your evenings won't feel quite as sharp.
Your mind won't fire as quickly.
Your body will soften a little sooner.
Your internal alarms won't go off at every quiet moment.
Your spikes of nighttime alertness will fade quicker.
Your mornings will feel more grounded.
Your nights will feel less like a fight and more like a natural transition.

These are the early signs that alignment is returning, not in dramatic leaps, but in steady, reliable steps.

Your nervous system is learning to trust again.

The Behavioral System in Motion

When you combine these anchors, morning rhythm, evening transition, nighttime ritual, and a safe bed, you create a behavioral environment where sleep becomes the natural response, not the forced goal.

And this is the key:

You are not teaching yourself to sleep.
You are teaching your body that it is allowed to.

Because when your systems feel safe, sleep becomes effortless.
What once felt impossible becomes instinct again.

This is where true realignment begins.
When your behaviors finally speak the language your body has been waiting

for, steady, predictable, reassuring, and your nervous system finally hears the message it forgot:

"You can rest now."

Section 2: Rebalancing the Biological System

The quiet physiology beneath your sleep, and how to realign it.

If the Behavioral System is the story you tell your body through your actions, then the Biological System is the story your body tells *you* through its chemistry, rhythms, and hidden processes.

Most people try to fix sleep by focusing on the mind, reducing stress, calming thoughts, "trying not to worry." But long before your mind gets involved, your biology has already shaped the night.

When your sleep fell apart, it wasn't just because you were busy or stressed. Your biological rhythms shifted. Your hormones learned the wrong timing. Your body adapted to unpredictability. And your physical systems began responding as if you were living in a low-level state of emergency, even when life had quieted down.

Rebalancing your biology doesn't require supplements or gadgets or a perfect routine. It requires giving your body the raw conditions it needs to trust the night again.

This section walks you back into biological alignment, gently, clearly, and in a way your body can respond to.

Where Biology Shows Up in Your Sleep

Your Biological System is built around a few key processes:

- **Your circadian rhythm**

- **Your sleep pressure system**

- **Your stress hormones**

- **Your temperature cycles**

- **Your light exposure patterns**

- **Your metabolic timing**

When these work together, sleep becomes effortless.
When they drift apart, everything feels unpredictable.

You know biology is misaligned when you experience:

- Tired but wired at night

- Sudden spikes of alertness

- Inability to fall asleep even when exhausted

- Feeling wide awake at 10 p.m. but crushed at 7 a.m.

- Waking up multiple times

- Feeling "electrified" at bedtime

- Not knowing when you'll feel tired

- Random bursts of energy late in the day

- Anxiety-like symptoms that are really biological misfires

These aren't flaws.
They're signals that your internal timing has drifted.

Your job now is to bring the system back into rhythm.

The Three Biological Forces You Must Realign

Sleep is largely determined by three biological processes.
Once you understand them, you stop blaming yourself and start working with
your biology instead of against it.

1. The Circadian Rhythm

Your internal clock, the anchor of your entire cycle.

You have a master clock in your brain that decides when you should be alert and when you should be winding down. It doesn't care how tired you are, it responds to:

- light

- temperature

- timing

- consistency

- patterns

When your circadian timing is off, you feel like your body is working against you. You can want sleep desperately yet not feel the biological "permission" to fall asleep.

You cannot negotiate with this clock.
You can only reset it.

This happens through two powerful cues:

- **Light exposure early in the day**

- **Evening dimness and gradual darkness**

These signals don't just help you wake up, they determine when melatonin releases at night. If your nights feel erratic, your circadian rhythm is crying for stability.

2. The Sleep Pressure System

The chemistry that builds your tiredness across the day.

There's a chemical called adenosine that slowly builds in your brain from the moment you wake up. The longer you're awake, the stronger it becomes, pushing your body toward deeper levels of fatigue.

But modern life interferes with this system:

- Late naps

- Caffeine too late in the day

- Inconsistent wake times

- Overstimulation

- Stress hormones blocking sleepiness

This creates a nighttime experience where you feel exhausted mentally but not physically ready to fall asleep. Sleep pressure hasn't accumulated the way it should.

To realign this system, you need steady wake timing, movement, and light exposure, the same tools used in the Behavioral System, now working on a deeper biological level.

3. The Stress-Arousal System

The most misunderstood biological force sabotaging sleep.

This is where most people get trapped.

Stress hormones like cortisol and adrenaline are designed to rise in the morning. But if your nervous system has been in survival mode for too long, these hormones shift, they release at the wrong times, at the wrong intensities, and in the wrong patterns.

You feel it as:

- racing thoughts

- tension in the chest

- pressure behind the eyes

- sudden alertness when you lie down

- jolting awake at 2 or 3 a.m.

- a surge of energy late in the day

- heart rate that won't settle

- "wired but tired" evenings

This isn't psychological, it's biological mis-timing.

When cortisol spikes at night or adrenaline remains elevated from the day, the body interprets it as a signal that shutting down might be unsafe.

Fixing this system isn't about calming down, it's about *helping your biology shift back into its proper timing.*
Your body settles when it believes it's safe, not when you try harder.

Bringing the Biological System Back Into Alignment

You cannot think your way into better sleep.
You must guide your body.

Here is how you realign the Biological System through gentle, reliable signals.

Restoring Circadian Timing

Give your internal clock the cues it needs.

Circadian rhythms are set by contrast: bright mornings, dim evenings.

Morning light:
Get outside or into bright light within the first hour of waking. This strengthens the wake signal and ensures melatonin will release at night.

Evening dimness:
Lower lights 2–3 hours before bed. This tells your brain the day is ending. Your melatonin release becomes stronger and more predictable.

Consistent wake time:
This is the most biologically powerful change you can make. Even after bad nights, waking at roughly the same time anchors your entire system.

This is why the Behavioral System matters, because biological realignment depends on behavioral predictability.

Restoring Sleep Pressure

Help your body rebuild natural tiredness.

Adenosine builds best when:

- you wake at the same time daily

- you avoid long or late naps

- caffeine is not consumed late in the day

- you move your body throughout the day

Movement is key, not heavy workouts, just steady activity. A slow walk, light stretching, household tasks. Each time you move, you're telling your body, "We are awake. Build pressure."

This is why people who sit all day often feel mentally tired but physically restless at night: sleep pressure never fully accumulates.

Lowering Nighttime Arousal

Let your stress hormones fall where they belong.

Cortisol and adrenaline need help coming down at night after years of being chronically elevated.

Several biological cues help:

Temperature drop:
Your core body temperature must fall to initiate sleep. A warm shower followed by cooler air helps the temperature shift your brain needs.

Sugar and heavy food timing:
Late heavy meals spike metabolic activity. Eat earlier when possible.

Stimulant reduction:
Caffeine has a half-life of 5–7 hours. Even an afternoon coffee can delay sleepiness.

Evening pacing:
Slow movement tells the nervous system, "There is no threat."

Predictable nights:
Biology responds best to rhythm. The more consistent your nighttime environment feels, the more your stress hormones settle.

This isn't relaxation, it's calibration.

The Invisible Rebuild

When your biology begins to realign, you may not notice it immediately. Instead, you notice subtle shifts:

- You start feeling waves of sleepiness at the right times.

- Your evening energy drops naturally instead of unpredictably.

- Your mind stops hijacking the night.

- Your awakenings become less dramatic.

- Your sleep feels deeper in certain pockets.

- Your mornings start feeling more grounded.

- Your body stops fighting you.

These changes are signs that your systems are synchronizing, that your biology is beginning to return to its natural arc.

You don't force this.
You create the conditions for it.

Once your Biological System stabilizes, the Emotional System becomes far easier to address because your body no longer interprets every quiet moment as a crisis.

This is the second system realigned.
And now your body is finally ready for the emotional repair that completes the transformation.

Section 3: Rebalancing the Emotional System

The weight you carry into the night, and how to finally release it.

If the Behavioral System shapes your patterns
and the Biological System shapes your rhythms,
then the Emotional System shapes your **experience of the night**.

This is the system most people blame themselves for.
This is the system almost no one understands.

Because the Behavioral System concerns what you do,
and the Biological System concerns how your body responds,
but the Emotional System concerns what you **feel** when everything gets quiet.

And that feeling, whatever it has become over the years, determines whether your nights feel like a place of rest or a place of reckoning.

For many people, nighttime becomes the moment their emotional load finally catches up to them. Not because they're weak or dramatic or anxious, but because the mind has been holding too much for too long. When the world goes still, your emotions rise. When distraction disappears, your deeper fears, pressures, and unresolved moments appear. When the house grows silent, your inner noise grows louder.

Sleep doesn't stand a chance until this system begins to soften.

Rebalancing the Emotional System isn't about forcing calm or shutting your thoughts off. It's about healing the relationship you have with the night, the part of your life where you're asked to let go, surrender control, and trust your body to take over.

For many people who've lived with stress or trauma or long seasons of responsibility, that surrender does not feel natural. It feels dangerous.

This is where we begin repairing that.

When the Night Stops Feeling Safe

You don't fear sleep, you fear the moment before it.
The quiet.
The stillness.
The space where everything unprocessed becomes impossible to ignore.

During the day, you're protected by distraction:
people, tasks, noise, deadlines, conversations, screens, motion.
Even if you feel overloaded, you're buffered by activity.

But at night?
The world shuts down.
Your mind does not.

It opens the drawers it kept closed all day.
It reveals the thoughts you didn't have time to think.
It surfaces the fears you didn't want to feel.
It replays the moments you didn't resolve.
It reminds you of everything you haven't yet handled.

This isn't anxiety.
This is an emotional backlog.

Your brain isn't malfunctioning, it's trying to do its job in the only time
you've given it to do it.

Understanding this releases the shame most people feel around nighttime
emotions. You are not broken. You are full, too full to settle.

Rebalancing this system is about helping your emotional load empty gradually,
instead of exploding at night.

Why Your Mind Activates the Moment You Lie Down

People often say, "I'm fine all day, but the moment I lie down everything hits
me."

Of course it does.

When you lie down, four things happen:

1. Your body signals "no more movement"
Your nervous system shifts from action to introspection.

2. Your external distractions disappear
No noise to drown out your internal world.

3. Your brain sees this as the only safe processing time
You're finally not performing, managing, or responding.

4. Your emotional load rises to the surface
Because it finally has room.

Your brain isn't attacking you, it's unloading you.
The problem is that it's trying to unload everything at once.

This is where emotional misalignment turns nights into battlegrounds.

The Hidden Emotional Load You Carry

Not all stress comes from "stressful events."
Most of it comes from micro-stress, small emotional hits that pile up throughout the day:

- the comment that bothered you but you ignored

- the task you didn't finish

- the responsibility you're holding

- the moment you felt unseen

- the pressure you put on yourself

- the fear of repeating last night

- the worry about tomorrow's demands

- the fatigue you don't want anyone to notice

Each of these is a drop.
One drop is nothing.
Hundreds form weight.

This is why you feel heavier at night, your Emotional System has no pressure valve during the day, so it releases everything at once when you finally stop moving.

This is not a flaw, it's physiology.
And it's fixable.

The Three Emotional Drivers You Must Realign

There are three emotional forces that determine whether your nights feel safe or charged:

1. **Safety**, your brain must believe nothing is required of you

2. **Permission**, your mind must feel allowed to release control

3. **Release**, your emotional load must have somewhere to go

When these three shift, sleep becomes possible again.

Let's walk through each one.

Restoring Emotional Safety

Teaching your brain that nighttime does not equal threat.

Your mind cannot let you fall asleep if it believes danger, emotional or imagined, might surface. This is why people who've endured stress, loss, transitions, uncertainty, or long-term pressure often struggle with sleep years after the stressor is gone.

The body healed.
The environment changed.
But the Emotional System never updated its programming.

It still believes night = vulnerability.

We reverse that through small, subtle acts of safety:

- Surround yourself with warm, gentle light

- Make your room feel comforting, not clinical

- Avoid conversations that spike emotion before bed

- Give yourself permission to get up without shame

- Let your evening routine feel nurturing, not obligatory

- Stop treating the bed like a test

- Speak to yourself with softness instead of pressure

Your brain responds not to logic, but to tone.

When your nights become "soft" instead of "urgent," emotional safety takes root again.

Restoring Emotional Permission

Removing the pressure to perform sleep.

Emotional permission is the antidote to nighttime fear.

Most people who struggle with sleep carry a silent rulebook:

- "I must fall asleep quickly."

- "I must handle tomorrow."

- "I must not fail again."

- "I must not feel anxious."

- "I must stay still."

- "I must control my mind."

Every "must" becomes emotional activation.
Every expectation becomes a threat.

Your mind interprets pressure as danger, even if the pressure is only about sleep.

Permission breaks that loop:

- "I don't have to force anything."

- "If I'm awake, I'm awake, and that's okay."

- "Thoughts are allowed."

- "Emotions are allowed."

- "My only job is to rest, not to perform."

Once you remove the emotional demand from the night, your nervous system begins to uncoil.

Sleep often follows not because you tried, but because you finally stopped trying.

Restoring Emotional Release

Letting the day come out of your body before the night begins.

Until your emotions have somewhere to go, they will go to the night.

Release doesn't mean unpacking your life story or reliving your trauma. It means giving your emotional system an outlet so the mind doesn't assume it must handle everything the moment you lie down.

A simple nightly release ritual helps clear the backlog:

1. Write the three heaviest thoughts from the day.
This tells your mind: "These won't be forgotten."

2. Name the emotion beneath them.
A single word is enough.

3. Write one thing you handled well.
This restores emotional balance.

4. End with a sentence of permission.
"I'm allowed to rest tonight."

Your emotional system responds to acknowledgment.
Once it feels heard, it stops shouting.

What Emotional Realignment Feels Like

People often report changes they didn't expect:

- The night stops feeling heavy

- Bedtime becomes less tense

- Thoughts feel quieter, less sharp

- Waking up at night becomes less dramatic

- Fear of the night fades

- The mind softens its edge

- Sleep comes in without being chased

- The body feels safer than before

This is not just sleep improving,
this is **you** improving.

Your Emotional System isn't something to battle.
It's something to comfort.
Something to understand.
Something to care for.

And when you do, sleep arrives naturally, not because you forced yourself to
be calm, but because your internal world finally feels safe enough to let go.

This is the final realignment.
This is where the weight leaves your body.
This is where the night belongs to you again.

Section 4: Bringing the Systems Back Into Harmony

Where your patterns, rhythms, and emotions finally meet again.

When your sleep first began to unravel, it probably didn't happen in one dramatic moment. It was gradual, a silent drift. A tightening here, a late night there, a season of stress that lasted longer than expected. One day you woke up and realized you couldn't recognize your nights anymore.

But that unraveling didn't mean you were broken.
It meant your systems were no longer moving together.

Your Behavioral System was sending mixed signals.
Your Biological System was receiving poor timing.
Your Emotional System was carrying too much weight.

Sleep became the casualty of misalignment, not the cause.

Now, for the first time in a long time, these systems are beginning to come back into harmony. You're rebuilding the very structure your body relies on to rest. You're giving your nights a shape again. You're teaching your biology timing again. You're showing your emotions they don't have to fear the dark anymore.

And something begins to shift inside you.

The Pattern Returns

As your Behavioral System stabilizes, you start moving through your days with a gentle predictability, not rigid, not perfectionistic, just steady. Your body learns where the day begins and where it ends. Your nights begin to feel less like a cliff and more like a path.

You may not notice the change immediately, but the people around you will.
Your evenings feel calmer.
Your pace softens.
Your mind isn't sprinting toward the next moment.

This is the first thread reweaving itself.

The Rhythm Returns

With each consistent morning, with each evening of dimness, with each night routine that unfolds in the same reassuring order, your biological rhythms start syncing again.

Your sleep pressure builds the way it's supposed to.
Your melatonin releases at the right time.
Your stress hormones fall into their natural arc.
Your temperature shifts exactly when it should.

Your body begins remembering its own design, the one it had long before your stress, your responsibilities, your traumas, your worries. The rhythm inside you was never lost; it was just drowned out by the noise of life. Now it's rising again.

You can feel it, a subtle pull toward rest, a natural heaviness at night, a gentle clarity in the morning.

This is the second thread stitching itself back into place.

The Safety Returns

As your Behavioral and Biological Systems strengthen their alignment, something sacred begins happening inside your Emotional System:
You stop bracing for the night.

You stop treating sleep like a test you're destined to fail.
You stop walking toward bedtime with fear in your chest.
The thoughts that once ambushed you lose their intensity.
The emotions that once spilled into the night find their place earlier in the day.

You start feeling like the night belongs to you again, not to your stress, not to your mind, not to your fears.

This is the deepest thread reconnecting, the thread of emotional safety.

When this thread returns, you no longer fight your mind.
You no longer fight your body.
You no longer fight yourself.

And in that absence of conflict, sleep returns naturally.

Your Systems Were Never Broken

When all three systems realign, your nights begin to follow a pattern that feels both new and familiar, new because it's been a long time, familiar because your body always knew how to do this.

This is the truth people rarely hear:

You were never "a bad sleeper."
Your systems were simply working with the conditions they had.

What looked like failure was survival.
What looked like anxiety was protection.
What looked like insomnia was adaptation.
What looked like chaos was your mind doing everything it could to keep you afloat during the hardest seasons of your life.

There was never something wrong with you.
There was only misalignment, and misalignment can be repaired.

You're doing that work right now.

A New Relationship With the Night

As your systems begin moving in harmony again, the night begins to change shape:

It stops feeling like a threat.
It stops feeling like a test.
It stops feeling like a place where your mind turns against you.

Instead, it becomes:

A return.
A release.
A steady exhale.
A reminder that rest is your right, not your reward.

This is what sleep feels like when your systems support you instead of fight you.

You don't have to try.
You don't have to force.
You don't have to control.
You just have to trust the alignment you're building.

Because now, the night is no longer where you struggle,
it's where you heal.

What Comes Next

Now that your systems are realigned, you're ready to move into the next phase of this journey, the part where you no longer just "fix" your sleep, but build the kind of sleep that strengthens your entire life:

Sleep that restores your mind.
Sleep that heals your stress.
Sleep that rebuilds your chemistry.
Sleep that gives you strength during the day.
Sleep that feels like a resource, not a battle.

In the next chapter, we step into the blueprint for sustainable, long-term alignment, the practices that make this transformation permanent, the patterns that keep your systems working together, and the lifestyle shifts that turn good nights into great ones.

You are no longer surviving the night.
You are learning to own it.

And from this point forward, sleep is no longer something withheld from you,
it becomes something you're finally ready to receive.

Chapter 10: The Night Transition Ritual

Section 1: The Dreameaz 60-Minute Wind-Down

How to guide your mind, body, and emotions into night with intention.

There is a moment each evening where your day stops, but your body doesn't. Your mind doesn't. Your nervous system doesn't. For years, you've likely moved through that moment without noticing it, pushing straight from activity to exhaustion, from motion to bed, from responsibility to stillness.

But sleep doesn't happen at the speed of your day.
Sleep happens at the speed of your **transition**.

The 60 minutes before you lie down form the most important hour of your night. This is where your systems either soften into alignment… or tighten into resistance. This hour decides whether your mind enters the night feeling supported or startled, whether your body flows toward sleep or fights it, whether your emotions settle or spill into the dark.

Most people don't have a nighttime problem, they have a **transition problem**.

The Dreameaz 60-Minute Wind-Down is built to repair that.
It's not a routine you perform, it's a ritual you enter.
A boundary between the world outside and the world inside.
A gentle descent from "doing" into "being."

This ritual is the bridge.
And tonight, for the first time, you'll cross it with intention.

Why the Final Hour Matters

Your nervous system doesn't care that you want to sleep, it cares whether it feels safe enough to. When your evenings carry the same pace, tone, and texture as your day, your system never receives the message that the "danger window" has closed.

This last hour tells your body:

- *The world is quiet now.*

- *Nothing else is required of you.*

- *You can stop holding everything.*

- *You can shift from performance to restoration.*

- *You can release.*

This ritual prepares your systems for the night the way a runway prepares an aircraft for flight, not with force, but with sequence.

And once your body learns that sequence, it begins anticipating sleep long before your head hits the pillow.

The Structure of the Dreameaz 60-Minute Wind-Down

This ritual unfolds in three gentle phases:

1. **Clearing the mental residue of the day**

2. **Softening the nervous system**

3. **Emotional grounding and release**

You move through them slowly, unhurried, allowing your systems to shift without pressure or performance. These phases are the physiological bridge into sleep, each one lowering a different kind of activation.

Let's begin with the first phase: Clearing the mental residue from the day.

Section 2: Clearing Mental Residue from the Day

Making space in your mind so the night doesn't have to hold everything.

The mind doesn't shut off at night because it's overactive, it shuts off because it's overloaded. All day long, you've been absorbing thoughts, decisions, moments, emotions, responsibilities, and unfinished loops. Most of them were small. Some were heavy. But all of them left a trace.

By the time evening arrives, your mind is still carrying the entire weight of the day. That weight becomes mental residue, the leftover fragments that didn't get processed fully, the invisible pressure of everything still unresolved, the "open tabs" your brain refuses to close.

If you don't clear this residue **before** the night begins, your mind will try to clear it **when** the night begins.

That's why people say:

- "My mind won't stop when I lie down."

- "Everything hits me at once."

- "I can't shut off."

Your mind is not malfunctioning.
It's trying to finish what the day didn't give it time to finish.

This part of the ritual gives your mind the space it needs to empty what it has been holding, gently, slowly, without digging or forcing or unpacking your entire life.

The goal is not to solve anything.
The goal is to release the mental weight you accumulated throughout the day.

The Three Forms of Daily Mental Residue

Your mind carries three types of "unfinished business" into the night:

1. Cognitive Residue

The tasks, decisions, and responsibilities you didn't complete:

- deadlines

- errands

- messages

- loose ends

- replayed conversations

- "don't forget" lists

These loops create cognitive pressure, which signals your brain to stay alert.

2. Emotional Residue

The subtle feelings you didn't process:

- frustration you pushed aside

- tension you ignored

- insecurity you buried

- overwhelm you disguised as productivity

- quiet sadness

- irritation you didn't want to deal with

Unprocessed emotion becomes nighttime activation.

3. Anticipatory Residue

The thoughts about tomorrow:

- "What if I'm tired?"

- "What if I can't sleep again?"

- "What if tomorrow becomes another disaster?"

- "Tomorrow is too much."

This residue keeps your brain in planning mode, the opposite of rest.

When you clear these three forms of residue *before* the night begins, you remove the mental fuel that keeps your mind awake.

The Dreameaz Clearing Ritual

This is a five-minute practice that empties the unnecessary weight from your mind.
It's simple. It's quiet. It's not "journaling."
It's unloading.

1. The Download

Write down anything your mind hasn't completed, tasks, thoughts, reminders, unresolved conversation fragments. Empty them onto a page or digital note.
This tells your brain: *"You don't have to hold this anymore."*

2. The Three Loops

Identify the three thoughts your brain keeps circling back to today.
Write them down exactly as they come.
This tells your brain: *"These are acknowledged."*

3. The Tomorrow Anchor

Write your top 1–3 priorities for tomorrow.
Not a full to-do list, just the anchors that matter.
This breaks anticipatory anxiety in half.

4. The Emotional Label

Name the strongest emotion you felt today, just one word.
Naming emotion reduces its activation by giving it identity.

5. The Permission Line

End with a simple sentence, spoken or written:
"I am done with today. I can rest now."

This closes the mental door the day left open.

Why This Works

Your brain hates open loops.
It loves conclusion.

When you externalize your thoughts, even briefly, the brain shifts out of problem-solving mode and into something softer, something closer to rest.

This five-minute release lowers cognitive arousal, reduces emotional intensity, and prepares your nervous system for the next phase of the transition: softening.

You don't need to feel "clear."
You just need to reduce the weight enough so your mind doesn't feel responsible for carrying the entire day into the night.

You're creating mental quiet, not through suppression, but through gentle release.

Section 3: Softening the Nervous System

The gentle descent from the pace of the day into the quiet the night requires.

Your nervous system is the bridge between your body and your mind.
It decides whether you're in "go mode" or "let go mode."
It doesn't speak in words, it speaks in signals.

All day, it's been absorbing noise, stimulation, decisions, expectations, stressors, micro-tensions, and subtle emotional hits. Even on a "good" day, your nervous system is performing on your behalf: keeping you alert, helping you focus, responding to challenges, managing surprises, adapting to the world around you.

By the time evening arrives, you're carrying the full pace of your day inside your body, often without realizing it. Your shoulders hold the tension. Your jaw holds the pressure. Your breath holds the speed. Your muscles hold the urgency. Your mind holds the momentum.

You cannot leap from that state into sleep.
Your body needs a *descent*.

Softening the nervous system is the second phase of the Dreameaz 60-Minute Wind-Down, and it is where your biology learns the truth:

"It's safe to stop."

Why Your Nervous System Fights the Night

When your nervous system is activated, it interprets stillness as vulnerability. It thinks:

- *"We're not ready to shut down yet."*

- *"We might need to act."*

- *"There's unfinished business."*

- *"Something could still demand my attention."*

This is not anxiety, **this is physiology.**

When your body is running on daytime activation:

- your heart rate sits slightly elevated

- your breathing remains shallow

- our muscles stay primed

- your thoughts stay fast

- your senses remain sharp

- your cortisol curve doesn't fall

- your body prepares for more "doing"

Sleep cannot begin in this state.
Your body must first be taught that evening is not a continuation of the day, it's a departure from it.

This phase teaches your nervous system how to cross that threshold.

The Descent Into Night

Softening doesn't happen instantly.
It happens through a sequence of physiological cues that tell your brain:

- slow down

- release tension

- lower vigilance

- quiet the inner motor

- dissolve the pace you carried all day

These cues speak to the parts of your nervous system that language cannot reach.

You're not calming yourself, you're recalibrating yourself.

The Dreameaz Softening Sequence

This part of the ritual focuses on three pillars: **pace, breath, and environment.**

Together, they work like a dimmer switch, lowering activation gradually until your body and mind meet in the same quiet place.

1. Slow Your Pace

Your nervous system mirrors your movement.
If your body moves quickly, your brain assumes urgency.
If your body moves slowly, your brain assumes safety.

For the next 15–20 minutes, move as though you are already halfway to sleep:

- walk slowly

- lower your voice

- soften your gestures

- reduce the speed of transitions

- let everything become unhurried

This isn't performance, it's signaling.

Your body listens.

2. Breathe Like the Night Has Already Begun

Your breath is the remote control for your nervous system.

During the day, you breathe quicker and higher in your chest. At night, your body needs slower, deeper, belly-led breathing, the kind that signals the parasympathetic nervous system ("rest and digest") to take over.

Try this pattern for a few minutes:

Inhale gently for 4 seconds
Exhale slowly for 6–8 seconds

The longer exhale tells your brain: *"We are not under threat."*

You don't need to meditate or concentrate.
Just breathe as though nothing urgent exists.

3. Shape Your Environment Into a Cocoon

Light, sound, and temperature all directly affect the nervous system.
Your environment becomes a language your body understands instantly.

Begin shaping your space for softness:

- lower lights

- switch from overhead lighting to lamps

- reduce volume, conversations, TV, music

- choose warm tones over bright ones

- lower room temperature slightly

- let the air feel cooler on your skin

- create a sense of warmth through blankets, textures, or scents

Your nervous system responds to contrast:
bright → dim
loud → soft
fast → slow
warm → cool
busy → calm

This contrast is what lowers activation.

Your body doesn't need silence, it needs gentleness.

What Softening Feels Like

It often begins quietly:

- your breath deepens

- your shoulders drop without you noticing

- your thoughts lose their edge

- your eyes feel heavier

- your inner pace slows

- your body feels grounded instead of braced

- your mind feels less like it's sprinting and more like it's strolling

- the night feels less threatening

- you begin to settle into your own presence

This is the nervous system shifting out of survival mode and into restoration mode.

Softening is *permission in physical form.*
It's your body remembering what safety feels like.

And when safety returns, sleep follows.

Section 4: Emotional Grounding Practices

Settling the emotional body so your mind no longer fights the night.

Once your thoughts have been cleared and your nervous system has begun to soften, there's one final layer that determines whether you cross fully into the night or hover at its edge: your **emotional state**.

Your emotional body is the part of you that carries tension, worry, memory, fear, hope, pressure, and expectation. It holds all the unspoken stories of your day, the things you didn't say, the feelings you didn't express, the disappointments you glossed over, the moments you rushed through.

The body remembers what the mind ignores.

If this emotional layer is unsettled, sleep becomes difficult even when the mind is quiet and the ody is tired. Emotional residue is lighter than mental residue, but more powerful. It doesn't shout, it hums. And that hum can keep you hovering just above sleep, unable to sink, unable to release.

Grounding is how you bring your emotional system back home.

This is not therapy.
It's not analysis.
It's not digging or forcing.

It's simply helping your emotional body feel safe enough to let the night have you.

The Emotional Body at Night

The emotional body responds to three states:

- **Uncertainty**

- **Unprocessed feelings**

- **Pressure**

At night, each of these becomes amplified.
The quiet feels too quiet.

The dark feels too revealing.
Your thoughts feel too close.

Grounding creates a container, a safe, steady inner space, so your emotions stop spilling into your night and instead settle where they belong.

The Dreameaz Emotional Grounding Method

This part of the ritual uses **three grounding practices**, each designed to anchor a different layer of your emotional system.

You only need one.
But many people combine them naturally over time.

1. The Weighted Exhale

A signal to the emotional body that it can finally let go.

The emotional system is deeply tied to the breath.
When emotions are activated, the breath becomes sharp, shallow, tight. When emotions soften, the breath becomes heavier and slower.

The Weighted Exhale uses the natural rhythm of the emotional nervous system:

- five slow breaths

- exhale slightly louder or heavier than the inhale

- allow your shoulders to fall each time

This sends a clear emotional signal:
You're allowed to stop holding everything.

You'll often feel a physical shift, a heaviness in the chest, a warmth behind the eyes, a settling in the body. That's emotional release.

2. The Hand Over Heart

A biological gesture that tells your emotional brain it's safe.

There's a reason people instinctively place a hand over their chest when overwhelmed. The emotional brain responds to **self-contact** as if someone is comforting you, because on a nervous-system level, it is.

Place a hand over your heart or the center of your chest.
Don't try to "feel calm."
Just stay there.

This gesture communicates reassurance to the emotional body:

- "I'm here."

- "You're safe."

- "You don't have to carry this alone anymore."

Within a minute or two, your emotional arousal drops.
Your nervous system shifts further into rest.
Your body begins preparing for surrender.

3. The 30-Second Naming

The simple act of acknowledging what you feel so your emotions don't spill into the night.

Emotions grow louder when ignored and quieter when named.

You don't need journaling.
You don't need explanation.
You don't need to solve anything.

Just name what you feel:

- "I'm carrying stress from the day."

- "I'm feeling a little sad."

- "I'm tired and overwhelmed."

- "I'm worried about tomorrow."

- "I'm feeling pressure."

A single sentence can release emotional tension that your body has been clenching tightly for hours.

This is not emotional analysis, it's emotional honesty.

Your brain hears the truth, and the emotional system finally softens.

When Emotional Grounding Works

You know grounding has begun when you feel:

- a softening behind the sternum

- a loosening in the jaw

- warmth in the chest or stomach

- a sense of space around your thoughts

- a drop in urgency

- a feeling that you could fall into bed rather than crawl toward it

- your mind reducing its grip

- your emotions settling instead of swirling

- the night feeling safe again

This is not "relaxation."
This is emotional alignment, the final phase before sleep.

The Completion of the 60-Minute Ritual

With your mind emptied, your nervous system softened, and your emotions grounded, your body enters the night already halfway into sleep's embrace.

You're not forcing anything.
You're not trying to sleep.
You're not battling thoughts.
You're not wrestling with tension.
You're simply transitioning, the way human bodies were designed to.

This hour becomes less of a routine and more of a sanctuary, a gentle, nightly return to yourself.

When these three layers settle together:

- cognitive

- physiological

- emotional

your body receives a message it hasn't heard in a long time:

"You can let go now."

And that's when sleep begins, not as a struggle, but as a natural descent.

The Completion of the Night Transition Ritual

Where your systems meet the night in harmony.

When you move through the Dreameaz 60-Minute Wind-Down, clearing the day from your mind, softening your nervous system, grounding your emotional world, something remarkable begins to happen beneath the surface.

Your systems stop working against each other.
They begin working **with** each other.

Your Behavioral System signals predictability.
Your Biological System responds with timing.
Your Emotional System settles into safety.

And for the first time in a long time, your mind, body, and emotions enter the night carrying the same message:

"Nothing is required of me now."

That is the state sleep needs.
That is the state we've been building toward.
That is the doorway into true rest.

When this ritual becomes part of your evenings, your nights stop feeling like a cliff you're trying to leap over. They become a slope, a gentle descent, where every minute brings you closer to the natural resting point your body has been craving.

This ritual is not about perfection.
It's not about checking boxes.
It's not about doing everything "right."

It's about creating the conditions where your systems can let go, where your brain no longer braces for the night, where your body no longer fights the process, where your emotions no longer overflow in the quiet.

This hour becomes your sanctuary.
Your separation from the noise of the world.
Your return to yourself.

And once your nights begin with intention, the architecture of your days begins to shift as well.

Because when you end each day grounded, clear, and supported…
you don't just sleep better,
you **live** better.

In the next chapter, we take everything you've learned and move into the long-term blueprint:
how to build a life, rhythm, and identity that keep your sleep aligned not just for weeks, but for years.

The night is no longer something you fear.
It's something you now know how to enter, gently, confidently, and whole.

Chapter 11: Falling Asleep, Staying Asleep, and Waking Well

Section 1: Why Effort Backfires at Night

The moment you start trying, your body starts waking up, here's why.

There's a moment in every struggling sleeper's night that feels almost sacred in its frustration. You've brushed your teeth, dimmed the lights, maybe even followed a perfect wind-down ritual. You're tired, desperately tired, and you think, *"Okay, this is it. Tonight has to work."*

You lie down.

You exhale.

And then, quietly at first, you begin the process every insomniac knows too well:

You start *trying*.

Trying to get comfortable.
Trying to stop thinking.
Trying to relax your body.
Trying not to check the clock.
Trying to breathe evenly.
Trying to sleep.

Trying.
Trying.
Trying.

But with every tiny effort, every micro-adjustment, every forced breath, every internal command, something inside you awakens. It's subtle at first. A little tension in the chest. A flicker of alertness behind the eyes. A mental tightening.

And then you feel it:

Sleep is slipping away.

The harder you try, the more awake you become.

It feels like betrayal, as if your own mind is working against you. But what's happening isn't betrayal at all.

It's biology.
It's survival.
It's your body doing exactly what it was built to do.

You're not broken, you're misunderstood.

Your Body Doesn't Understand "Trying to Sleep"

Effort is a daytime tool.
During the day, effort solves problems. Effort gets things done. Effort helps you perform, respond, and protect yourself.

But at night, effort sends the wrong message to your nervous system.

To your body, effort means:

- alertness

- attention

- vigilance

- monitoring

- danger

- threat

Effort means you need to stay awake.

You lie there trying to fall asleep, but your nervous system hears that effort and thinks:

"Something important is happening."

Those tiny adjustments?
Your body reads them as preparation.

Those forced deep breaths?
Your brain reads them as regulation, something people do under pressure.

That mental monitoring, *"Am I asleep yet?"*, sends another signal of vigilance.

And the more vigilant you become, the more your sympathetic nervous system engages, the system designed to keep you alive, not asleep.

Sleep isn't something the brain *executes*.
It's something the brain *allows* when it feels safe.

Effort equals danger.
Danger equals wakefulness.

And suddenly the equation makes sense.

The Moment Night Becomes a Performance

There is a very specific moment when sleep stops being natural and becomes performance. It's the moment when the night becomes a test, a challenge, a measurement of your worth or competence or strength.

You feel it when you think:

- "I can't mess this up."

- "I have to sleep tonight."

- "Tomorrow depends on this."

- "Please… just work."

- "I can't afford another bad night."

This is where the emotional system gets entangled with the biological one. Because those thoughts don't just live in your mind, they live in your chest, your breath, your heart rate, your hormones.

Performance pressure turns sleep into danger.

Your body goes on alert not because you're dramatic, but because alertness is what kept your ancestors alive. Your brain doesn't know the difference between a tiger and a presentation tomorrow morning. All it senses is urgency.

Urgency is the enemy of sleep.

Why Sleep Slips Away the Moment You Reach for It

Sleep is a doorway you walk through, not one you push open.

The harder you push, the more it closes.

Trying to sleep is like trying to fall in love on command, or trying to feel inspired on cue. It's not a task, it's a state.
And states cannot be forced.
They must be entered.

Your biology has a very simple rule:

Anything you track, you wake up for.

Track your breaths?
You wake up a little.

Track your comfort?
You wake up a little.

Track your thoughts?
You wake up a little.

Track time?
You wake up a lot.

Sleep doesn't want your attention, it wants your absence.

A Story Every Sleeper Knows

Imagine lying in bed after a long day. Your body is tired, but your mind is hovering, alert, calculating, trying to figure out what position, what breath pattern, what exact internal state might finally "unlock" sleep.

You tell yourself:
"Just relax."

But the moment you command relaxation, your brain starts scanning to see if it's working.

That scan wakes you further.

You try to breathe deeply.

The effort turns your breathing into a task, and now your mind is supervising it.

You try to clear your thoughts.

The act of noticing a thought makes you more aware of it.

You turn over.

Your nervous system interprets the movement as readiness, not rest.

You open your eyes.

The room feels off.

You close your eyes again.

Your heart beats harder.

You think, *"Not again."*

And now you're fully awake.

Not because you "failed."

But because you "tried."

The Shift That Changes Everything

There is one sentence that shifts your entire relationship with sleep:

"It's not my job to sleep. It's my job to allow the conditions where sleep can happen."

This is the core of the Dreameaz method.

You remove effort.
You remove pressure.
You remove performance.

And in that space, sleep returns, not because you earned it, not because you forced it, but because you finally stepped out of the way.

Your systems know what to do.
Your biology knows what to do.
Your emotional body knows what to do.

They just need you to stop trying and start allowing.

Section 2: Release → Reset → Re-Enter

A three-part process for falling asleep and returning to sleep without fear or effort.

Once you understand that effort backfires, you need something else, a sequence that replaces effort with rhythm, pressure with permission, and panic with direction.

That's what **Release → Reset → Re-Enter** is.

It is the Dreameaz nighttime cycle, the method you'll use whether:

- you're lying down and can't fall asleep

- you wake up at 2 a.m.

- your mind feels sharp

- your chest feels tight

- you feel "wired" instead of tired

- you fear the night repeating itself

Most people stay stuck because they don't know what to *do* when sleep doesn't come. They lie in bed frozen, hoping the moment will pass, or spiraling deeper into urgency. They wait, worry, overthink, monitor, and try to force sleep into happening.

You're about to learn a different way, one that keeps your nervous system regulated, your emotional system grounded, and your confidence intact.

The Core Problem: Staying in Bed Too Long When Awake

One of the biggest mistakes struggling sleepers make is staying in bed while awake and uncomfortable.
This trains your brain to associate your bed with:

- stress

- tension

- desperation

- endless thinking

- helplessness

- fear

The longer you lie there trying to sleep, the stronger this association becomes.

Release → Reset → Re-Enter breaks this cycle by giving you a **structured, compassionate way out**, and a way back in.

You're no longer trapped.
You're guided.

This is what your nights have been missing.

THE SYSTEM

1. RELEASE

Step out of the pressure so your system stops escalating.

Release means the moment you notice:

- you're trying to sleep

- you're uncomfortable

- your mind won't settle

- your chest feels tight

- you're starting to spiral

- you're becoming too alert

…you **release the attempt.**
Not by trying harder to relax, but by stopping the performance of sleep entirely.

Release is the moment you say:

- "Okay. I'm awake right now."

- "Nothing is wrong."

- "My job is not to force anything."

- "This is just a moment."

Then you **get out of bed gently.**

Not dramatically.
Not angrily.
Not panicked.
Just softly.

Like you're stepping out to stretch.

You don't need to leave the bedroom.
You just need to change your position, your environment, and your mental state.

Release ends the fight.
It tells your brain:

"No danger here. We're okay."

This alone prevents 90% of nighttime spirals.

2. RESET

Shift your nervous system and emotional body out of activation.

Once you've stepped away from the bed, you move into the reset.
This is the most important part of the entire cycle.

Reset doesn't mean you try to get sleepy.
Reset means you help your body return to its baseline.

You choose one gentle activity from a short menu, something calming, grounding, and non-stimulating:

- sit in a dim room

- do slow breathing (4 in, 6 out)

- read a neutral book

- stretch lightly

- place a hand over your heart

- hold a warm mug

- sit by a window in the dark

- listen to calming background noise

The rule is simple:

**If it raises your heart rate or engages your mind, it's too stimulating.
If it numbs or distracts you aggressively, it's too harsh.
Reset should feel like softening, not escaping.**

This part of the cycle tells your nervous system:

"We're safe again. The pressure is gone."

Your emotional body uncoils.
Your cortisol begins to fall.
Your system starts drifting toward rest on its own.

Reset can last 5–20 minutes.
You don't time it.
You feel it.

You know you're ready for the next step when your internal pace slows down.

3. RE-ENTER

Return to bed only when the body, not the mind, invites you back.

You re-enter the bed the same way you'd re-enter a warm room you stepped out of for a moment, gently, naturally, without pressure.

The key is this:

You only return when your body feels softer and your nervous system has shifted out of alert mode.

You're not returning because:

- "It's been long enough."

- "I should try again."

- "I need to sleep."

You return because:

- your breath is slower

- your thoughts feel less sharp

- your chest feels less tight

- your pace feels gentler

- your body feels ready to settle

This is when your biology is actually able to receive sleep.

When you lie back down, you don't "try again."
You simply enter the bed as if you're entering rest, not performing sleep.

If sleep comes, it comes.
If not, you run the cycle again.

Why This Works

Release → Reset → Re-Enter works because it:

- breaks the association between bed and struggle

- interrupts the panic that forms when you stay in bed too long

- prevents your nervous system from escalating

- reinforces the bed as a place of safety

- gives your brain clear, reliable structure

- removes the fear of "What do I do if I can't sleep?"

- returns control to you without creating pressure

- respects your biology instead of fighting it

You are no longer trapped with your thoughts.
You are no longer stuck in the bed.
You are no longer hostage to the night.

You have a process.
And that process keeps your systems aligned even when sleep doesn't happen immediately.

This cycle becomes your nighttime anchor, the way you navigate the night with confidence instead of fear.

Section 3: Breaking Nocturnal Panic

How to stop the fear spiral that turns a single moment of alertness into a full night of suffering.

Nocturnal panic is one of the most terrifying experiences a struggling sleeper can face. It's the moment when a normal awakening, something every human experiences multiple times a night, turns into a surge of adrenaline, a racing heart, a flood of thoughts, and a wave of helplessness.

It can feel like the night is swallowing you whole.

But what's really happening is simpler, more human, and far less dangerous than it feels.

Breaking nocturnal panic is not about getting rid of fear, it's about understanding it so intimately that its power over you dissolves.

The Anatomy of Nocturnal Panic

Nocturnal panic has a predictable sequence.
Knowing this sequence is how you regain control.

1. A neutral awakening

You wake up, sometimes to reposition, sometimes spontaneously. This is normal. It happens to everyone.

2. Unexpected alertness

For a split second, you feel more awake than you expected.
Your brain reacts: *"Why am I awake? What's wrong?"*

3. A tiny spark of fear

It's barely noticeable, but your body registers it.
This spark triggers a quick release of adrenaline.

4. The spike

Your heart rate increases.
Your breath tightens.
Your chest feels warm or hollow.
Your stomach drops.
Your mind jumps to attention.

5. Catastrophic interpretation

Your thoughts begin racing:

- "It's happening again."

- "Not tonight."

- "I won't be able to sleep."

- "Tomorrow will be ruined."

- "I can't do this."

6. Full activation

Your nervous system shifts into a sympathetic state, the fight-or-flight system.

This is the moment where you feel trapped in your own body, unable to fall asleep, unable to calm down, unable to stop the spiral.

But here's the truth:

Nothing here is dangerous.
Nothing here is permanent.
Nothing here means you're broken.

Your body is simply misinterpreting the night.

And you are about to learn how to correct that misinterpretation.

The Core Misunderstanding: Fear of the Fear

Most people think the panic itself is the problem.
It's not.
The panic is a brief physiological surge that *always* passes.

The real problem is the fear of the panic, the mental interpretation that something catastrophic is happening.

When you fear the fear, your panic becomes a loop:

Sensation → Interpretation → Fear → More Sensation → More Fear

Your body isn't panicking because something is wrong.
It's panicking because it thinks you need protecting.

Your only job is to help your system recognize that the night is safe again.

Breaking the Panic Loop

There are three steps to interrupting nocturnal panic in real time.
These steps work not by suppressing the panic, but by dissolving the signal that keeps feeding it.

1. Name the Sensation

This removes its power.

Say to yourself, silently or out loud:

- "This is a surge."

- "My nervous system woke up."

- "My body thinks I need protection."

- "This is temporary."

Naming the sensation shifts your brain from emotional interpretation to factual recognition.
You cannot panic and observe at the same time, observation wins.

2. Ground the Body, Not the Mind

Trying to calm your thoughts only amplifies them.
Instead, calm the body, and the mind will follow.

Use one of these grounding cues:

- place a hand on your chest

- sit up and plant your feet on the floor

- take one slow exhale longer than your inhale

- relax your jaw

- drop your shoulders

These actions interrupt the sympathetic surge and signal safety.

3. Leave the Bed with Confidence

This is the moment you use Release → Reset → Re-Enter.

At the first sign of panic escalation, you **leave the bed gently**, not out of fear but out of strategy.

This action breaks the association between:

- bed ↔ fear

- bed ↔ panic

- bed ↔ helplessness

By stepping away, you reset the environment, reduce the panic, and prevent the bed from becoming the stage where panic rehearses itself.

You are not escaping the panic.
You are interrupting its pattern.

And when patterns break, panic dissolves.

What Happens When You Stop Feeding the Panic

When you respond to nocturnal panic with structure instead of fear:

- the panic loses its intensity

- the spike shortens

- the night becomes manageable

- awakenings become neutral again

- confidence replaces dread

- panic stops returning night after night

You stop fearing the night.
And when the fear dissolves, the panic loses its oxygen.

Your nervous system learns:
"This is not danger. This is just noise."

Once the fear of the fear disappears, nocturnal panic never returns in the same way.

The Most Important Realization

Nocturnal panic is not a sign of weakness.
It is not trauma resurfacing.
It is not your mind betraying you.
It is not your body malfunctioning.

It is a **misinterpreted surge**, a signal without a threat.

And once your brain learns to interpret the night differently, the surges stop turning into storms.

You reclaim your nights not by stopping panic…
but by understanding it so clearly that it finally releases you.

Section 4: Temperature & Cortisol Control

How two quiet biological forces can make or break your night, and how to use them wisely.

If you've ever been on the edge of sleep and suddenly felt wide awake for no reason…
If you've ever jolted awake in the middle of the night with a racing mind…
If you've ever felt "wired" when you should feel exhausted…
If you've ever wondered why some nights your body feels electric…

You've experienced the work of two powerful biological players:

Temperature and cortisol.

These two forces control more of your nighttime experience than most people realize. When they rise or fall at the wrong time, your body misinterprets the night. But when they align properly, they support one of the most effortless sleep descents you've ever felt.

And the best part?
They are two of the easiest systems to influence, once you understand how they work.

The Temperature Rule: You Can't Sleep Until You Cool

Your core body temperature must **drop** in order for sleep to happen.
This is non-negotiable biology.

Think of it like this:

During the day, your internal temperature stays slightly elevated to support alertness. When night comes, your body attempts to drop its core temperature to begin the cascade into sleep.

This drop signals:

- melatonin release

- lowered arousal

- muscle softening

- heart rate calming

- slowed brain activity

- readiness for surrender

But here's the problem:

Modern life often **traps us in too much heat** before bed, showers that are too hot, rooms that are too warm, blankets that are too heavy, screens that stimulate, movement that generates heat, even emotional activation that warms the chest.

When your core temperature can't fall, your brain concludes:

"It's not night yet. Stay awake."

This is why some people feel wide awake after a hot shower.
Why some feel alert under too many blankets.
Why others toss and turn in a warm room.

Your body is trying to cool, and failing.

How to Use Temperature to Your Advantage

Small shifts make a big difference:

1. Use the Warm-to-Cool Drop

Take a warm (not hot) shower 60–90 minutes before bed.
Warm increases surface blood flow.
Stepping into cooler air afterward triggers the necessary drop.

2. Keep Your Bedroom Cooler Than You Think

Ideal sleep temperature: **60–67°F (15–19°C)**
Cool air signals safety and rest.

3. Use Layers, Not Heavy Heat

Light layers let your body regulate on its own.
Heavy bedding traps heat and blocks the nightly temperature drop.

4. Uncover Your Feet

Your feet help regulate body heat.
When they're uncovered, your core cools quicker.

5. Avoid late-night workouts

Exercise raises core temperature for hours.
A late workout can push your sleep window back.

Your body wants to cool.
Help it, don't fight it.

Now, the Other Half: Cortisol

The engine behind nighttime alertness.

Cortisol is often misunderstood.
It's not the "enemy hormone."
It's your activation hormone, the one that helps you wake up, think clearly, and take action.

But when cortisol spikes at the wrong time, the night becomes a place of tension instead of rest.

A nighttime cortisol spike feels like:

- sudden alertness

- racing mind

- heart rate rising

- chest pressure

- internal buzzing

- feeling "too awake"

- mild anxiety out of nowhere

- difficulty falling back asleep

You've probably blamed your thoughts for this.
But what you're really feeling…
is chemistry.

Why Cortisol Spikes at Night

1. Stress carried too late into the evening

Your emotional system didn't have a release valve.

2. Stimulating activity late at night

Even small tasks can elevate arousal.

3. Overthinking or planning in bed

Your brain interprets cognitive load as daytime activity.

4. Blood sugar dips

This triggers adrenaline, which triggers cortisol.

5. Waking up suddenly

The brain sometimes over-corrects with alertness.

6. The fear of not sleeping

Fear is a cortisol activator.

Cortisol spikes are not sabotage, they are misread signals of urgency.

Rebalancing Nighttime Cortisol

Just like temperature, stabilizing cortisol is about rhythm and gentle signals:

1. Dim Lights = Lower Cortisol

Light, especially overhead or white-blue light, prevents your cortisol from falling.
Warm light helps it drop.

2. Slow Your Pace

Fast movement = daytime.
Slow movement = nighttime.
Your nervous system mirrors your pacing.

3. Soften Your Breath

Exhaling slower than you inhale signals safety.
Safety lowers cortisol.

4. No clocks

Clock-watching spikes cortisol through fear and urgency.

5. Gentle carbohydrates in the evening

Not sugar, small, balanced carbs.
This stabilizes blood sugar and prevents adrenaline spikes.

6. Release → Reset → Re-Enter

The cycle prevents your cortisol from turning a basic awakening into full activation.

As cortisol falls, the night stops feeling sharp.
Your internal world stops buzzing.
Your system becomes receptive again.

When Temperature and Cortisol Align

When your core temperature drops
and your cortisol curve begins its natural descent,

you feel it.

It's the unmistakable sensation of your body surrendering:

- warmth moving out of the chest

- heaviness settling into your limbs

- breath deepening

- thoughts losing their edges

- senses softening

- an internal gravity pulling you downward

This is the descent into sleep,
not forced, not chased, but **allowed.**

Temperature and cortisol don't just influence sleep.
They *invite* it.

And learning to work with them, rather than stumbling into misalignment,
gives you one of the most powerful tools for falling asleep and getting back to
sleep effortlessly.

Section 5: The 3AM Rescue Protocol

*What to do when the night wakes you, and how to prevent a single awakening from
becoming a full-night battle.*

There is something uniquely fragile about 3 a.m.

Not 9 p.m.
Not midnight.
3 a.m.

It's the hour where your inner world feels louder, your outer world feels
emptier, and every thought feels heavier than it should. You're awake, but not
fully. Aware, but not grounded. Your mind is active, but it's thinking with half
its power and twice its emotion.

You are in what psychologists call a **hypnagogic vulnerability window**, a
state where your emotional centers are far more active than your logical ones.
This means:

- small worries feel enormous

- neutral sensations feel threatening

- thoughts feel sticky

- emotions feel unfiltered

- your body feels exposed

- your sense of control feels thin

It's not your fault.
It's not a malfunction.
It's just what the 3 a.m. hour does to the human brain.

This section teaches you how to navigate this hour without fear, without spiraling, and without losing your night.

This is the Dreameaz **3AM Rescue Protocol**, your step-by-step map through the darkest moment of the night.

Why 3AM Feels Different

When you wake at 3 a.m., your brain is in **Stage 1 sleep physiology**:

- cortisol is naturally at its lowest

- emotional centers are unusually active

- rational centers are partially offline

- body temperature is at its minimum

- nervous system is more sensitive

- thoughts are easily distorted

- time perception becomes warped

Your brain is literally designed to be *less stable* at this hour.
That's why:

A small spike feels like a panic attack.
A normal awakening feels like danger.

A simple thought feels like a spiral.
A mild sensation feels like something is wrong.

Your brain is not trying to hurt you, it's trying to protect you with the limited tools it has available in that moment.

The Rescue Protocol corrects that misinterpretation.

The Four-Stage Rescue Protocol

1. Pause & Recognize the State

This is not full wakefulness, it's a transition.

The first 10 seconds after waking are the most important.
This is where panic either blooms or dissolves.

Instead of going into:

- "Why am I awake?"

- "Not again."

- "Here we go…"

- "Tomorrow's ruined."

You say something simple and grounding:

"This is a half-wake state. It always passes."

A half-wake state means:

- your emotional brain is louder

- your logical brain is dimmer

- nothing you think right now is accurate

- your sensations are exaggerated

- your mind is not in problem-solving mode

You're not *awake*, you're *in between*.

Recognizing this strips the fear of its power.

You're waking into a state that will stabilize on its own, as long as you don't panic.

2. Breathe Down the Surge

The panic spike loses steam when your exhale takes the lead.

When you wake suddenly, or with anxiety, you're often feeling a sympathetic nervous system micro-surge, a short burst of adrenaline meant to check the environment for danger.

It's a harmless reflex.

But if you interpret it as danger, your fear adds more fuel.

The fix is simple:

Inhale 4 seconds
Exhale 6–8 seconds

No counting.
No "deep breathing" effort.
Just slow, heavier exhaling.

Why?

Because the long exhale directly communicates with the vagus nerve, the switch that calms your heart rate, slows your fear response, and tells your amygdala (your alarm center):

"False alarm. Stand down."

Within 30–60 seconds, the spike begins to loosen:

- heartbeat slows

- chest pressure releases

- thoughts lose their sharpness

- the "electric" feeling fades

You're not calming yourself, you're recalibrating.

3. Leave the Bed Before the Spiral Hooks You

The moment you feel the escalation begin, you interrupt it.

Staying in bed while awake is what turns a moment into a nightmare.

If you lie there thinking:

- "Just relax…"

- "Come on…"

- "Why now…"

- "It's okay, it's okay…"

…your brain begins associating your bed with stress.

This creates the bed-panic loop.

So instead, you do something counterintuitive but transformative:

You get out of bed gently.

Not angrily.
Not dramatically.
Not in defeat.
Just softly, like stepping out of a warm bath for a moment.

This breaks the neurological pairing:
bed = panic
bed = alertness

The body can reset once the environment resets.

This step alone prevents long nights of spiraling.

4. Reset With Grounded Neutrality

You're not trying to sleep, you're letting the chemistry settle.

Now that you're out of the bed, the goal is not to "get sleepy."

The goal is to return your nervous system to its baseline.

Choose one neutral, grounding activity:

- sit in a dim room with soft light

- place a hand on your chest

- breathe slowly and naturally

- read a few pages of something neutral

- listen to soft, non-engaging sound

- sip warm (non-caffeinated) tea

- stare out a window into the dark

- stretch very lightly

Nothing stimulating.
Nothing goal-oriented.
Nothing that feels like you're "trying to fix this."

What you're doing is letting the cortisol dip continue and allowing your temperature curve to settle.

After 5–20 minutes, you'll feel a shift:

- your mind stops racing

- your chest softens

- your breath deepens

- your body feels heavier

- the emotional fog clears

Only then do you return to bed.

What Happens When You Return to Bed

Re-enter the bed like you're returning to warmth, not to perform, not to test yourself, not to "try again."

Simply lie down, soften your body, and let the bed hold you.

If sleep returns, good.

If it doesn't, you're not stuck.
You simply run the cycle again.

Confidence replaces panic.
Process replaces fear.
Structure replaces helplessness.

Your body learns:
"Waking up is not a threat."

And once the fear dissolves, the awakenings lose their bite.

The Hidden Victory: You Break the Fear of the Night

The real transformation here isn't that you fall back asleep faster, though you will.

The real transformation is:

- the fear collapses

- the anticipatory dread disappears

- the night loses its sharpness

- the awakenings stop being emotional

- your confidence returns

- your body stops bracing

- sleep becomes safe again

You no longer think, "I hope I don't wake up tonight."

You think, "Even if I do, I know exactly what to do."

That mindset alone is enough to change someone's life.

This is the beginning of reclaiming the night forever.

Section 6: Morning Reset and Energy Calibration

How to begin the day in a way that protects your night, even after a rough sleep.

Most people think their night determines their day.
But for great sleepers, it's actually the other way around:

Your day determines your night.

How you wake, how you move through the first ninety minutes of the morning, and how you regulate your energy throughout the day create the conditions your body will use that night.

If your morning begins in panic, rushing, self-judgment, or compensation for "not sleeping enough," your nervous system stays elevated all day, and elevated systems do not descend easily when night comes.

Morning is not just waking up.
Morning is **resetting your biology** for the next 24 hours.

This section teaches you exactly how to do that.

The First Rule of Mornings: The Night is Over

Whether you slept poorly…
or beautifully…
or somewhere in between…

The night ends the moment you wake with intention.

You are not analyzing the night.
You are not measuring it.
You are not checking the clock.
You are not reviewing the "failures."
You are not replaying your awakenings.

All of that drags the identity of "struggling sleeper" into the next day.

The first words you tell yourself set the emotional tone:

"This day is mine. The night is over."

This shift protects your nervous system from carrying nighttime fear into the morning.

Your night does not get to define you.
Your morning will.

The Morning Reset Sequence

Your morning reset has three phases:

- Light

- Movement

- Direction

These recalibrate your circadian rhythm, cortisol curve, energy curve, and mental stability for the rest of the day.

Let's break them down.

1. LIGHT: Anchor the Clock

Light is the single strongest regulator of your circadian rhythm.

Within 10–30 minutes of waking, sooner if you can, you want **natural outdoor light** in your eyes.

Not sunglasses.
Not through a window.
Actual daylight.

Why?

Natural morning light triggers:

- a healthy cortisol rise (the good kind)

- a predictable 14–16 hour sleep countdown

- increased daytime alertness

- stabilized mood

- stronger sleep drive at night

- better nighttime melatonin release

Even on cloudy days, natural light is 5–10x stronger than indoor lighting.

Aim for 2–10 minutes outdoors.
More if it feels good.

This is how you tell your brain:
"It's daytime. Build energy now. Rest later."

2. MOVEMENT: Signal the Shift Into Wakefulness

Your body wakes in layers.
Your mind might be up, but your biology is still shaking off the night.

Movement finishes the transition.

This does **not** mean a full workout.
It means:

- walking

- stretching

- joint mobility

- gentle yoga

- light activity

Even a few minutes of movement:

- increases circulation

- stabilizes cortisol

- reduces sleep inertia

- improves clarity

- builds natural energy

Movement tells the body to rise, not through adrenaline, but through rhythm.

This protects you from the morning grogginess spiral that leads to caffeine overload and nighttime disruption.

3. DIRECTION: Give Your Mind a Gentle Anchor

When you wake after poor sleep, your mind often wants to catastrophize:

- "Today is ruined."

- "I won't function."

- "Everything will be harder."

- "I can't keep doing this."

These thoughts activate the emotional system and create a cortisol spike that shadows your entire day.

The fix is not positive thinking.
The fix is **direction.**

Give your mind the next small step, nothing more.

Examples:

- "Make coffee."

- "Take a shower."

- "Get outside for light."

- "Walk the dog."

- "Open the blinds."

When the mind is given a direction, it stops searching for threats.

This anchors your emotional system and stabilizes your morning energy.

How to Handle Grogginess Without Ruining Your Day

Grogginess is not failure.
It's chemistry.

You treat it gently:

- hydrate early

- avoid caffeine in the first 30–60 minutes (to avoid cortisol interference)

- choose light movement

- expose yourself to natural light

- avoid lying back down

- avoid slow emotional rumination

Your job is not to eliminate grogginess.
Your job is to prevent it from controlling the tone of your day.

When grogginess is handled well, it fades.
When grogginess is feared, it intensifies.

Avoiding the Two Major Traps That Destroy Your Night

Trap 1: Overcompensation

After a poor night, you might be tempted to:

- nap
- sleep in
- skip your morning routine
- reduce activity
- cancel plans
- drink extra caffeine
- conserve energy

These actions delay your circadian timing and make the next night worse.

You don't punish yourself, but you don't collapse your structure either.

You simply move through the day gently, without extremes.

Trap 2: Storytelling

The biggest destroyer of sleep is the daytime story:

- "I can't function on poor sleep."
- "I'm exhausted."
- "Why does this always happen?"
- "I'm going to crash tonight."

These thoughts keep your nervous system elevated all day, and nothing elevated during the day easily descends at night.

Morning is where you break the story.

Energy Calibration Throughout the Day

Your goal during the day is not to maximize energy.
Your goal is to **stabilize** it.

This keeps your nighttime systems stable.

1. Break the day into energy zones

- Morning = activation

- Afternoon = steady engagement

- Evening = softening and descent

2. Avoid the afternoon crash trap

A large crash leads to late-day caffeine, naps, or overeating, all of which disrupt circadian timing.

Use movement, hydration, and natural light to stay stable.

3. Keep emotional spikes low

If something stressful happens, regulate early:

- slow breath

- brief pause

- mental labeling

- physical grounding

This prevents cortisol from staying elevated into the evening.

Why This Matters for Sleep

Morning is where your body decides:

- how much sleep pressure to build

- how predictable your rhythm will be

- how smooth your cortisol curve will look

- how stable your emotions will be

- how easily you can descend at night

A well-calibrated morning protects you from nighttime chaos.

A chaotic morning creates nighttime vulnerability.

Your night doesn't begin at bedtime.
Your night begins when you wake.

And with the Morning Reset sequence, Light, Movement, Direction, you protect your night before it even begins.

The Emotional Shift That Changes Everything

Imperfect nights don't ruin you anymore.

Because now you know:

- how to handle them

- how to support yourself

- how to stabilize your day

- how to protect your evening

- how to fall asleep

- how to return to sleep

- how to wake well

You are no longer at the mercy of your nights.
You're leading them.

And when your days and nights support each other, sleep stops feeling fragile, it becomes a natural rhythm again.

Chapter 12: Living a Sleep-Positive Life

Section 1: Staying Steady Through Chaos and Change

How to keep your sleep stable when life stops playing by the rules.

There's a version of sleep that works only when life is calm, when your schedule is predictable, your emotions are steady, and your routines unfold the way you planned.
That kind of sleep is fragile. It breaks the moment reality shifts.

What you're building now is different.
What you're building is **sleep that survives real life**, sleep that stays intact when everything around you changes.

To do that, you need two things woven together:

1. **Your foundational anchors, the non-negotiables you already learned.**

2. **Your chaos frameworks, the tools that reinforce those anchors when life gets loud.**

This chapter is where those two worlds meet.

Why Chaos Affects Sleep So Deeply

Chaos doesn't disrupt sleep because you're weak or unprepared.
Chaos disrupts sleep because it destabilizes three systems at once:

- **your biological rhythms**

- **your emotional load**

- **your behavioral predictability**

When these three wobble, even slightly, sleep becomes vulnerable.

This is why people who are making progress often panic during stressful weeks.
They think they're "slipping back," when in reality, their systems simply lost stability.

Sleep doesn't need perfection.
It needs grounding.

That's where your anchors come in.

Your Three Anchors, Revisited as Lifelong Stabilizers

Earlier in the book, we built your anchors:

- predictable wake time

- protected morning

- gentle nighttime descent

They were introduced as tools.
Now, they become **identity-level stabilizers.**

You don't have to remember a list.
You don't have to perform them perfectly.
You don't even need them to be long or elaborate.

You just need them to exist, consistently, even in small forms.

Anchor 1: The Wake-Time Rhythm

Not rigidness.
Not punishment.
Just rhythm.

Waking within the same window stabilizes your internal clock, even in messy seasons.

Anchor 2: The Morning Reset Signal

You don't have to "win the morning."
You just need:

- a bit of light

- a bit of movement

- a bit of direction

This resets your biology after chaotic nights.

Anchor 3: The Nighttime Descent Line

Your wind-down can shrink during difficult times,
but it should never disappear.

Even 10 minutes of softening your pace signals your body that the day is
ending.

These anchors form the **backbone** of permanent sleep.
But chaos requires more than a spine, it requires flexibility.

This is where the new layer comes in.

The Chaos Compatibility Model™

The reinforcement system that keeps the anchors strong during crisis, stress, upheaval, or emotional turbulence.

When life becomes unpredictable, emotionally, physically, professionally, your
anchors need extra reinforcement.
Not more technique… just more support.

The Chaos Compatibility Model has **three stabilizers**:

Stabilizer 1: Containment

Protecting your emotional system from flooding the entire night.

Containment is not suppression.
It's the ability to say:

**"This emotion is allowed, but it does not control the tempo of my
evening."**

Containment practices include:

- mini check-ins

- naming emotions without analysis

- brief grounding

- safe conversations

- controlled venting

This prevents the emotional system from hijacking your anchors.

Stabilizer 2: Pacing

Maintaining internal speed even when your external world accelerates.

During chaos, your body speeds up automatically.
Your thoughts move faster.
Your movements become sharper.
Your decisions become reactive.

Pacing slows the internal tempo so your anchor points still have space to work.

Pacing looks like:

- intentionally slowing physical movement

- gentle transitions

- micro-pauses throughout the day

- reducing multitasking

- creating "breathing pockets" in stressful hours

This keeps your biological rhythms from spiraling.

Stabilizer 3: Preservation

Protecting the small habits that keep your systems stable, even when everything else is lost.

This is the heart of the Chaos Compatibility Model.

Preservation means:

- You don't try to do everything.

- You don't try to maintain the whole routine.

- You don't aim for perfect alignment.

You just preserve the **minimum effective dose** of the anchors.

This turns your sleep plan into something that bends without breaking.

How Anchors + Chaos Compatibility Create Permanent Sleep

Anchors create stability.
Chaos Compatibility creates resilience.

Together they produce:

- nights that don't collapse during stress

- nervous systems that don't spin out

- identity shifts that hold even under pressure

- a relationship with sleep that feels grounded, not fragile

You no longer depend on calm circumstances.
You no longer fear unpredictability.
You no longer lose your progress when life gets loud.

You become someone who sleeps not because life is easy…
but because you know how to stay anchored through difficulty.

This is what makes your sleep plan permanent.

Section 2: Calming PTSD Episodes

How to navigate trauma-driven nights without fear, collapse, or losing control of your sleep.

There is a unique kind of night that trauma creates, a night that doesn't behave like other nights.
A night where your body remembers things your mind wants to forget.
A night where old memories arrive uninvited, triggered by small moments, thoughts, sensations, or sometimes nothing at all.

This is the night where you wake up sweating, or shaking, or confused.
The night where your heart is sprinting but your body can't move.
The night where the room feels unfamiliar, too dark, too quiet, too sharp.
The night where your mind floods with images that don't belong to the present moment.

If this is part of your story, understand something clearly:

**Your trauma reacts at night not because you're fragile…
but because the night is when your defenses are down.**

PTSD episodes at night aren't a sign that you're broken.
They're a sign that your body is still trying to protect you with the only language it learned during survival.

This section teaches you how to calm those episodes without fear…
so you can sleep even when your history tries to wake you.

Why PTSD Shows Up Strongest at Night

Nighttime is fertile soil for past pain because:

1. The world gets quiet

Your brain loses distractions.
Old memories find space.

2. Your emotional brain is more active

At night, the amygdala (your fear center) increases activity, while your logical cortex goes partially offline.

3. Your nervous system loses its "day armor"

You're no longer in motion, no longer braced, no longer distracted.
Stillness reveals what movement hides.

4. Darkness triggers ancestral vigilance

Your brain is wired to scan for danger in the dark, especially a brain
conditioned by trauma.

This combination creates nighttime vulnerability, not because you're weak,
but because biology becomes more reflective and less defensive under quiet.

But vulnerability does not mean danger.
Not anymore.

Understanding the PTSD Night wave

A PTSD episode at night has a recognizable pattern.
When you know it, you can interrupt it.

1. The Trigger

It might be:

- a sound

- a dream

- a memory fragment

- a physical sensation

- an emotional residue from the day

- or nothing at all

Triggers don't need logic. They only need association.

2. The Body Responds First

Your heart rate spikes.
Your breath locks.

Your muscles tighten.
Heat floods your chest or face.
Your stomach drops.
Your limbs feel heavy or unreal.
Your senses sharpen.

This is your survival system taking over.

3. The Mind Interprets

Suddenly, you're not just awake, you're in a different time, a different place, inside an old story your body still thinks is happening.

The mind doesn't think in words here.
It thinks in images, emotions, and alarm.

4. The Identity Collapses

This is the hardest part.
You feel transported, not literally, but emotionally.

You feel like:

- the past is happening again

- you're losing control

- you're unsafe in your own body

- you've gone backward

- you're failing

But this moment is survivable.
And with the right process, it becomes reclaimable.

The PTSD Night-Calming Framework™

A four-part system to navigate trauma-triggered awakenings without spiraling.

This framework helps your body reorient to the present moment, your mind returns to safety, and your emotional system settles enough for sleep to re-enter.

1. Orientation

Remind your nervous system where you actually are.

The first step isn't breath,
it's **place.**

When trauma wakes you, the brain temporarily loses orientation, thinking you're back inside the memory's environment.

You restore orientation through simple, grounding statements:

- "This is my room."

- "This is my bed."

- "I'm safe now."

- "That was a memory, not a moment."

- "This is my present."

You can also orient physically:

- touch the sheets

- press your palm to the mattress

- look at a familiar object

- feel your toes wiggle

- sit up slowly

This tells the fear center:
**"We are not there.
We are here."**

2. Containment

Bring the emotional surge into a manageable window.

Containment doesn't mean pushing feelings down.
It means creating edges around them, so they don't overwhelm your system.

Try:

- placing a hand on your chest

- naming the emotion: "fear," "anger," "sadness," "shock"

- reminding yourself: "This is intensity, not danger."

- speaking one grounding sentence: "I can feel this safely."

Containment reduces emotional flooding by 30–50% within minutes.

It helps your body understand:
"This does not control me."

3. Co-Regulation (Even Alone)

Using external cues to stabilize an internal storm.

Trauma dysregulates the nervous system.
Co-regulation brings it back.

If you're with someone you trust:

- ask for physical presence

- a hand on your back

- grounding words

- rhythmic breath together

If you're alone:

- listen to a calming voice recording

- use soft music

- wrap yourself in a blanket

- hold something weighted

- sit against a wall for grounding pressure

Your body doesn't need a person,
it needs **something predictable** to regulate against.

Predictability equals safety.

4. Descent

Guide your system downward, slowly, without force.

Once your fear center is less activated, your goal is not to "go back to sleep."
Your goal is to descend.

Descent can look like:

- slow breathing

- rocking gently

- stretching the hands and feet

- moving your jaw to release tension

- repeating a grounding phrase

- stepping out of bed for 2–3 minutes

Once the emotional wave has crested and softened, you re-enter the bed
gently, not to sleep, but to settle.

Sleep returns naturally when the trauma wave loses steam.

The Most Important Promise

A PTSD episode does **not** erase your progress.
It does **not** restart your sleep journey.
It does **not** mean your body is broken.
It does **not** mean your trauma is "back."
It does **not** mean the night is lost.

It means you're human.
It means a memory got activated.
It means your body is still healing.

And the fact that you know how to calm yourself through it…

That is the definition of recovery.

You no longer fear the night.
You no longer fear your body.
You no longer fear the memories that once controlled you.

You've learned to carry yourself through the dark without collapsing inside it.

This is how you build a sleep life that is **trauma-informed, resilient, and permanent.**

Section 3: Managing High-Performance Seasons

How to protect your sleep when life asks you to be more than human.

There are stretches in life when you don't get the luxury of slowing down.
Not because you don't want to, but because something bigger is pulling you forward.

It might be a goal you've waited years to chase.
A promotion that demands the best of you.
A season in your career where the stakes rise.
A project you cannot let fail.
A competition you're preparing for.
A role only you can fill.
A crisis only you can manage.
A window of opportunity you refuse to miss.

These are not normal weeks or normal months.
These are **becoming seasons**, the ones that forge you, define you, and demand pieces of you that the rest of the world will never see.

And it's during these seasons that sleep becomes most at risk.

Not because you don't care about your well-being…
but because your entire system shifts into a mode you learned young:

"I'll push through."
"I'll handle it."
"I'll collapse when it's over."

High performers rarely burn out because they're weak.
They burn out because for too long, they were *strong in the wrong places*, in their drive, in their pace, in their ability to suppress their limits.

They forget that even excellence has a nervous system attached.

The Silent Drift Away from Sleep

High-performance seasons don't steal your sleep all at once.
They erode it quietly.

At first, you feel energized, sharper than normal, fueled by purpose.
Your mind is loud in a good way, ideas firing like electricity.

But gradually, something shifts:

1. Your days get longer, but your decompression gets shorter.

You finish late and jump straight into the next thing.
You tell yourself you'll slow down tomorrow.

Tomorrow never arrives.

2. Your nervous system never fully returns to baseline.

You stay half-activated, even during dinner, even while brushing your teeth, even when your head hits the pillow.

3. Your pace becomes your identity.

You stop noticing the speed you're living at.
You start believing this is just "how you perform."

4. Your body gets addicted to the adrenaline drip.

You feel powerful…
until the lights go out.

And that's when the cost shows up.

You lie down, but your mind keeps its foot on the gas.
Your body tries to cool, but your cortisol refuses to fall.
Your chest stays a little tight.
Your breath stays a little shallow.
Your thoughts keep rehearsing tomorrow.

You're tired, but your system doesn't know how to stop.

High performance didn't break your sleep.
It just replaced your descent with momentum.

The Moment You Realize Your Engine Has No Brake

There's a night, every high performer knows this one, where you lie in bed
and realize something unsettling:

You don't feel tired anymore. You feel charged.

Your body hums like it's still mid-day.
Your mind feels like it could keep working for hours.
Your legs feel restless.
Your thoughts jump from idea to idea.
You're physically exhausted… but internally *awake*.

This is not insomnia.
This is **over-performance physiology.**

Your body has confused productivity with survival.

Your brain is saying:

- "We're in the middle of something important."

- "Stay sharp."

- "Stay ready."

- "Not yet. Not now."

Your biology thinks you're in the middle of a hunt, not the end of a day.

High performers don't need to learn how to sleep.
They need to learn how to *stop*.

And stopping, for people wired like you, feels harder than anything you accomplished during the day.

The Quiet Truth: If You Don't Create an Off-Switch, You Don't Have One

When life accelerates, most people respond by sacrificing the soft moments:

- You shorten your wind-down.

- You answer "just one more" email.

- You eat later, move less, push harder.

- You carry the day's pressure straight into the night.

- You stop listening to your body because you're listening to your goals.

And then you hit a wall that doesn't look like burnout, it looks like:

- racing thoughts

- midnight awakenings

- your heart beating faster than it should

- the "wired-tired" feeling

- restless legs

- sharp alertness at 2 a.m.

- crashing mid-afternoon

- a mind that won't descend

The truth is simple:

High performance without recovery is just slow collapse.

But you don't need to give up your ambition.
You don't need to soften your drive.

You just need to support the biology that supports the ambition.

The Performance Preservation Framework

A narrative model for staying excellent without losing yourself.

This isn't a list of rules.
This is a way of living inside high-performance seasons without sacrificing your nervous system.

It has three components, not techniques, but **reorientations**.

1. Micro-Descent: Teaching Your System to Pause Before You Fall

High performers don't need more rest, they need more *edges* between tasks.

Instead of running your day like one continuous sprint, you create small, controlled descents.

These aren't breaks.
These are *interruptions to momentum*:

- a single slow breath before you open your laptop

- pausing your body for two seconds between emails

- walking instead of rushing

- releasing your shoulders before a meeting

- lowering your voice right before you speak

- moving your jaw to release tension

- turning your face toward natural light for five seconds

These micro-descent moments tell your nervous system:

"We are not in danger. You don't have to stay elevated."

This stops adrenaline from stacking.
It prevents the nightly crash.
It teaches your physiology that performance is not threat.

2. Boundary Bookends: The First and Last 10 Minutes

When you can't control the whole day,
you control the edges of it.

Even in your busiest seasons, you can protect:

The first 10 minutes after waking

- natural light

- breath

- movement

- orientation

This stabilizes your adrenaline curve so it doesn't stay elevated all day.

The last 10 minutes before bed

- dim lights

- slow breaths

- softened pace

- emotional release

This signals your brain that the day has actually ended.

Ten minutes.
Not perfection, transition.

These bookends aren't rituals.
They're circuit breakers.

3. The Enough Point: Redefining What Completion Means

High performers often finish their day emotionally unfinished, carrying loops, tasks, worried thoughts, pressure.

This keeps the system in "continuation mode."

The Enough Point is the moment you decide:

"The rest can live until tomorrow."

You draw a soft line between the day and the night, not by completing everything, but by releasing everything that didn't get done.

You don't descend because the tasks end.
You descend because you *stop carrying them*.

The Enough Point is what prevents nighttime reactivation.

The Identity Shift of the High Performer Who Sleeps

Something changes when a high performer finally realizes:

"My performance is only as strong as my recovery."

You stop treating sleep as interference.
You start treating sleep as infrastructure.

You stop treating rest as downtime.
You start treating it as preparation.

You stop measuring success by exhaustion.
You start measuring it by capacity.

And eventually, this becomes your internal truth:

**"I don't sleep less during high-performance seasons,
I protect my sleep more."**

Because you know what it costs when you don't.

This is how high performers evolve into sustainable performers.
Not softer.
Not slower.
Just longer-lasting, more grounded, more powerful versions of themselves.

This is what secures your sleep for life, even when life demands more than usual.

Section 4: The Dreameaz 7-Day Recalibration Protocol

Your one-week reset for getting back in rhythm, without pressure, punishment, or perfection.

Every sleep journey has drift.
Even the strongest sleepers slip out of rhythm sometimes.
A stressful week.
A tough month.
A painful season.
A few bad nights that turn into a pattern.
A storm of responsibilities that disrupts everything.

Most people panic when they fall out of sync.
They think:

- "I'm slipping back."

- "It's happening again."

- "I lost all my progress."

- "I'm starting over."

254

But progress in sleep, real progress, is not measured by never drifting. It's measured by how easily and confidently you can **return to center**.

That's what the Dreameaz 7-Day Recalibration Protocol is for.
It's not punishment.
It's not correction.
It's not "starting over."

It's the **homecoming week**, the week where you reconnect with your rhythm, reset your systems, and rebuild confidence in your body's ability to sleep.

This protocol is short, gentle, and powerful.

It works because it aligns your behavioral, biological, and emotional systems all at once.

Why a 7-Day Reset Works So Well

Seven days is enough time to:

- realign your circadian timing

- stabilize your cortisol curve

- rebuild sleep pressure

- re-establish evening descent

- remove fear from awakenings

- calm your emotional system

- re-anchor your identity as a good sleeper

But it's *not* long enough to:

- feel intimidating

- require perfection

- overwhelm you

- create pressure

A week is long enough to change you
and short enough to not scare you.

This is what makes the recalibration protocol work.

How to Use This Week

Before we begin, understand one thing:

This is not a detox or a challenge.
This is a reset.
A recalibration.
A return.

If you miss a day, you continue.
If you skip something, you return when you can.
If you wake up at 3 a.m., the protocol absorbs it.
If life gets messy, the protocol bends.

This week is not here to judge you.
It's here to hold you.

Now let's begin.

DAY 1, The Reset Signal

"My week starts here."

Day 1 is about direction, not perfection.

Three things happen today:

1. You pick a consistent wake window.

Not a precise minute, a *window*.
This creates stability without rigidity.

2. You do the Morning Reset (light, movement, direction).

This stabilizes your cortisol rhythm immediately.

3. You do a 10-minute wind-down.

Not a full ritual, a transition.

Day 1 tells your body:
"We're shifting back."

DAY 2, Rebuilding the Rhythm

Let your systems feel the pattern again.

Today you repeat the three Day 1 actions.
But you add one more piece:

4. A micro-descent break every 3–4 hours.

Just 10–20 seconds of slowing your breath or pace.

You're resetting your daytime tempo
so your nighttime descent is easier.

Your body begins to remember the slope of the day.

DAY 3, Deepening Safety

Calming the emotional system.

On Day 3, you add a simple evening practice:

5. A 2-minute emotional release.

This can be:

- naming your strongest emotion

- talking it out

- writing a few lines

- long exhale breathing

- hand over heart

This step alone reduces nighttime activation.

Tonight feels easier.

DAY 4, Clearing Residue

Lightening the load your mind carries into bed.

This is the day you reintroduce the mental clearing practice.

6. The 3-minute thought download

You offload:

- unfinished tasks

- looping thoughts

- tomorrow's priorities

- mental pressure

This clears space in your head for the wind-down to work.

Your system begins to trust the night again.

DAY 5, Strengthening the Descent

Rebuilding your nighttime slope.

Tonight you extend your wind-down to 15–20 minutes.

Not heavy.
Not complicated.
Just slightly longer and more spacious.

You soften:

- light

- movement

- breath

- emotional tone

Your body begins relearning how to surrender.

You feel the difference immediately.

DAY 6, Normalizing Awakening

Healing your relationship with the middle of the night.

Today, you practice the mindset shift:

7. "If I wake, I handle it."

You rehearse, mentally, the Release → Reset → Re-Enter cycle.
Not because you expect to need it…
but because knowing you can use it removes the fear that keeps you awake.

Confidence is what prevents spirals.

Tonight feels like freedom.

DAY 7, The Identity Day

The day where the shift becomes who you are again.

The final day of the recalibration protocol is not about behavior.
It's about identity.

You end the week by anchoring yourself back into the truth:

"I am someone whose body knows how to sleep."
"I am someone who can return to rhythm easily."
"I am someone who is safe at night."

You reflect, briefly, on how much gentler the week felt.
You notice how different your mind feels about sleep.

You notice how aligned your systems feel.
You feel the weight lifting.

By Day 7, you're not forcing sleep.
You're allowing it.

The reset is complete.

When to Use the Recalibration Protocol

Use it when:

- you drift

- you have a chaotic week

- you come back from travel

- you have PTSD flare-ups

- you enter a high-performance cycle

- you go through emotional turmoil

- sleep feels "off"

- you feel disconnected from your routines

- you just need to reconnect with your rhythm

You don't wait for a crisis.
You use it to prevent one.

Section 5: Building Environments and Relationships That Protect Rest

Sleep is not just something your body does.
It's something your *life* allows.
Or doesn't allow.

Long-lasting sleep doesn't come from hacks or supplements or short-term wins.

It comes from shaping a world around you that finally says:

**"You can stop now.
You're allowed to rest."**

This world isn't built overnight.
It's built choice by choice, relationship by relationship, boundary by boundary, breath by breath.
And most people don't even realize they're living inside a world that keeps their body awake, not because of danger, but because of *unresolved responsibility, tangled emotions, and unspoken expectations.*

Sleep cannot flourish in a life that constantly demands your alertness.

So as you step into the final stretch of this journey, I want you to see your sleep not as a nightly event,
but as something your entire world is conspiring to protect.

Or working against.

Let's rewrite that world.

Your Environment Tells a Story About Who You've Become

Walk into your bedroom tonight and notice what it says about you.

Every object, every light, every noise, every habit…

…is telling your nervous system a story.

- "There's still work to finish."

- "This room is chaotic."

- "This home isn't peaceful."

- "You're responsible for everything."

- "You can't slow down yet."

But your environment can also tell a *very* different story:

- "You're safe here."

- "You've done enough for today."

- "This is your quiet place."

- "The world can wait outside this room."

- "You are allowed to surrender."

When you soften your world...
your world softens you.

This is what reshapes your nights.

Not perfection.
Permission.

A Supportive Environment Doesn't Need Luxury, It Needs Intention

People think that better sleep requires a perfect bedroom.
It doesn't.

It requires a bedroom that understands you.

A space that:

- doesn't yell at your senses

- doesn't pull your attention

- doesn't remind you of your to-do list

- doesn't activate tension or memory

- doesn't demand anything of you

You're creating a place where your nervous system can finally stop keeping score.

Sometimes the most powerful sleep improvement is not a mattress, or a supplement, or a gadget,

but simply removing the noise, clutter, or chaos that makes your body think it
still has to stay awake.

The room becomes a container for your descent.
A place that holds you while you let go.

That's not design.
That's healing.

The Relationships Around You Matter More Than You Think

Your sleep is shaped by more than the room you lie in.
It's shaped by the people you live alongside.

Human nervous systems are not solitary systems, they sync, co-regulate,
attune, and respond to the emotional energy of others.

The people close to you contribute to your nights in ways you don't see:

- a tone of voice

- a rushed evening

- the lack of emotional closure

- an unresolved argument

- someone's anxiety spilling into your space

- someone's expectations weighing your shoulders

- someone needing you when you're trying to descend

- someone moving quickly while you're trying to soften

This isn't about blame.
It's about recognition.

Your nights are deeply shaped by the emotional ecosystem you live in.

Better sleep does not require perfect relationships,
just *clearer* ones.

Clear expectations.
Clear communication.
Clear emotional boundaries.
Clear space to soften.

When your relationships begin to respect your rhythms, your sleep stops feeling like something you have to fight for,
and starts feeling like something the people around you want to protect.

The kind of sleep that lasts a lifetime is sleep supported by your world, not resisted by it.

The World You're Building Will Outlive This Book

This last section isn't really about environment or relationships.

It's about your life.

About creating a world where:

- your body no longer lives in defense

- your mind doesn't end each day in battle

- your emotional system has room to breathe

- your nights are not something you brace for

- your mornings don't feel like recovery from survival

- your sleep is not fragile because your life is not frantic

You're building a life that doesn't sabotage your biology.
A life that doesn't steal from your nights to pay for your days.
A life that doesn't constantly keep you alert.
A life that can hold you gently without needing you to hold everything.

And the truth you've earned, after all the chapters you've walked through, after all the nights you've survived, is this:

Your sleep becomes permanent when your life becomes safe for it.

Safe emotionally.
Safe environmentally.
Safe relationally.
Safe internally.

When you build a world that supports rest, sleep stops being something you chase,
and becomes something you naturally receive.

This is the final transformation of Chapter 14.
Not better nights.
A better life.

A life aligned with peace, permission, and protection.

A life where rest is not a struggle…
but a homecoming.

Conclusion: The Night You Come Home to Yourself

If you've reached this page, it means something important:

You didn't give up on yourself.

You walked through every chapter, the hard ones, the emotional ones, the uncomfortable ones, and you kept going. You looked at your nights honestly. You faced the parts of yourself you once avoided. You learned things about your body, your mind, and your life that most people never even realize matter.

And because you stayed with it, you are no longer the same person who began this book.

Your sleep is not the same either.

The Journey You've Just Walked

You didn't just learn techniques.
You learned a new way of understanding yourself.

You learned:

- how your days influence your nights

- how your biology speaks in rhythms

- how your emotions echo in the dark

- how misalignment, not brokenness, creates sleeplessness

- how to create safety, predictability, and descent inside your own life

You learned that sleep is not a battle.
It is a relationship.

And at every step of this journey, you proved something:

You were never the problem.
You were never "bad at sleeping."

You were simply unaligned, and alignment is something you can rebuild.

My Story Is the Proof That This Is Possible

I want to say something clearly, because it matters:

I didn't write this from a mountain looking down upon people who struggle.
I'm not a brain doctor.
I'm not a heart specialist.
I'm not a psychiatrist with a wall full of diplomas telling you how to fix something I've never experienced.

I am you.

I am your peer, someone who struggled for years with the same fears, the same sleepless nights, the same racing mind, the same anxiety spikes, the same 3 a.m. awakenings, the same emotional storms, the same desperate desire to feel normal again.

I didn't start as an expert.
I started as someone who was suffering.

And I realized something along the way that no doctor or sleep technician ever told me:

Most people who teach sleep have never truly fought for it.
They teach pieces of the puzzle, bits of research, fragments of theory, but they rarely understand the full lived experience. They see data, not desperation. They see symptoms, not stories.

I wanted something different.

So I became my own experiment, my own case study, my own patient, my own teacher. Through research, trial and error, setbacks, and breakthroughs, I began to see the whole puzzle clearly for the first time.

What you've read in this book is not theory.
It is the system I built from the inside, the system that saved my nights.

Today, I can say something I once thought I'd never be able to say again:

I am a better sleeper.

Not a perfect sleeper.
A *real* sleeper.

Someone who understands my triggers.
Someone who knows how to reset.
Someone who trusts my body again.
Someone who uses the tools in this book not because I'm fragile, but because they work.

And that's the point I want to leave you with:

Recovery isn't perfection.
Recovery is the ability to realign quickly.

That's what I learned.
That's what you've learned too.

Your Story Is Just Beginning

You now have the same tools I use.
The same understanding.
The same clarity.
The same roadmap.

You now know how to:

- protect your rhythm

- manage chaos

- calm your body

- soothe your emotions

- break panic cycles

- navigate trauma echoes

- reset your nights

- rebuild your mornings

- reconnect your systems

- reclaim your identity as a sleeper

You no longer depend on luck.
You no longer fear setbacks.
You no longer need someone else to "fix" you.

You have become your own expert, from the inside.

The Nights Ahead of You

There will still be imperfect nights.
That's part of being human.

But something is different now.

You won't spiral.
You won't fear the darkness.
You won't feel helpless.
You won't feel broken.
You won't feel alone inside your own experience.

Now, when a night feels off, you'll know exactly what to do:

Stop.
Observe.
Identify the misalignment.
Reset.
Re-enter.

This is the gift you've earned, the ability to return to yourself, again and again.

The Truth You Carry Forward

As you close this book, there is one truth I want you to carry with you:

Your body wants to sleep.
It always has.
It just needed a life, a rhythm, and a system that allowed it.

You've built that system.
You've built that life.
You've built that understanding.

Sleep is no longer a mystery.
It is no longer a threat.
It is no longer something you chase.

It is something you return to.

Something that belongs to you.

Something that has always belonged to you.

The night is yours again.

Welcome home.

Thank you for letting me walk this path with you, not as an expert, not as a doctor, but as someone who understands, who's lived it, and who believes in your ability to reclaim your nights.

I'm proud of you for making it this far.
I hope you're proud of yourself too.

Paul

APPENDIX A - THE DREAMEAZ SLEEP AUDIT

A foundational assessment for identifying misalignment across your Behavioral, Biological, and Emotional systems.

Before You Begin: A Short Note

This Sleep Audit is the **core, streamlined version** of the Dreameaz assessment. It gives you everything you need to understand your sleep patterns, uncover your biggest misalignments, and begin the realignment process described in this book.

However, this is the **light version**.

The full, 20–30 page **Dreameaz Comprehensive Sleep Diagnostic**, used in the Dreameaz Course and membership, includes:

- chronotype and circadian rhythm profiling

- cognitive activation mapping

- trauma-linked sleep pattern analysis

- nervous system regulation scoring

- emotional safety and nighttime triggers

- environment & sensory overstimulation audit

- relational co-regulation profile

- lifestyle pace & burnout index

- recovery capacity scoring

- misalignment archetype classification

- personalized alignment plan

If you ever want the complete diagnostic experience, you can access it at:

www.dreameaz.com

For now, the audit below is the perfect place to begin.

HOW TO USE THE SCORING MODEL

Throughout this assessment, you'll use a simple 1–10 scale:

1–3: Minimal Misalignment

Not a primary contributor to sleep disruption. Strong areas to build from.

4–6: Moderate Misalignment

Meaningful contributors. Improve these, and sleep improves quickly.

7–8: Significant Misalignment

Major drivers of nightly instability. High-impact targets.

9–10: Critical Misalignment

Core sleep breakers. Not signs of failure, signs of where alignment will create the most transformation.

This audit identifies patterns.
Patterns tell your story.
And stories can be rewritten.

THE DREAMEAZ SLEEP AUDIT

This audit is organized around the three systems discussed throughout the book:

- **Behavioral** (patterns, timing, habits)

- **Biological** (physiology, rhythm, activation)

- **Emotional** (stress, trauma, safety, load)

It also evaluates environment, lifestyle, cognitive activation, and recovery capacity, giving you a fuller picture of how your days shape your nights.

Take your time.
Breathe.
Be honest.

This audit is not about judgment.
It's about clarity.

SECTION 1, NIGHTTIME EXPERIENCE SNAPSHOT

Your lived experience of the night.

1.1 Sleep Continuity

- Number of awakenings per night: ____

- Typical wake time(s): ____________

- Body sensations during awakenings (check):
  ☐ heart racing
  ☐ overheated
  ☐ shaking
  ☐ restless legs
  ☐ numbness/tingling
  ☐ none

- Emotional tone of awakenings:
  ☐ calm ☐ anxious ☐ panicked ☐ disoriented ☐ sad ☐ alert

- Average duration awake: ____ minutes

1.2 Morning Experience

- First feeling when waking (check all):
  ☐ foggy ☐ wired ☐ tired but functional ☐ drained ☐ rested ☐ hopeful

- Typical wake time: ___________

- Do you snooze? ☐ Yes ☐ No

- Wake time varies more than 45 minutes? ☐ Yes ☐ No

SECTION 2, BEHAVIORAL SYSTEM AUDIT

Patterns, timing, routines, and structure.

2.1 Timing & Routines

- Consistent bedtime? ☐ Yes ☐ No

- Average bedtime: ___________

- Do you fight your bedtime when tired? ☐ Yes ☐ No

- Do you get a "second wind" at night? ☐ Yes ☐ No

2.2 Sleep Onset (1–10)

Rate the following:

- Difficulty falling asleep: ____

- Mind racing when lights go out: ____

- Physical tension (shoulders, jaw, chest): ____

- Emotional heaviness before bed: ____

- Using distraction (screens/TV/scrolling) to avoid silence: ____

- Fear or dread of bedtime: ____

2.3 Daytime Patterns (1–10)

Rate:

- Pace/intensity of your day: ____

- Transition ability (moving between tasks): ____

- Cognitive load (problem-solving, planning): ___

- Time spent multitasking: ___

- Emotional energy expended during day: ___

2.4 Evening Rhythm

- Average last meal time: ___________

- Caffeine after 3 pm? ☐ Yes ☐ No

- Exercise within 3 hours of bed? ☐ Yes ☐ No

- Evening social interactions energizing or draining?
  ☐ Energizing ☐ Draining ☐ Neutral

2.5 Behavioral Sleep Breakers (check all that apply)

☐ late eating
☐ late work
☐ night-time responsibilities
☐ screens in bed
☐ chaotic evenings
☐ emotionally heavy nights
☐ unpredictable schedule
☐ rapid task-switching near bed

SECTION 3, BIOLOGICAL SYSTEM AUDIT

Physiology, activation, and rhythm.

3.1 Physiological Activation (1–10)

Rate:

- muscle tension baseline: ___

- chest tightness: ___

- jaw clenching: ____

- restlessness at night: ____

- overheating: ____

- heart rate spikes: ____

3.2 Circadian Rhythm Clarity

Check any patterns:

- ☐ difficulty feeling sleepy at night

- ☐ alertness spike after 9 p.m.

- ☐ morning grogginess

- ☐ inconsistent hunger cues

- ☐ irregular bowel rhythm

- ☐ afternoon crash

- ☐ late-night energy

3.3 Biological Influencers

- Caffeine sensitivity (1–10): ____

- Alcohol impact on sleep (1–10): ____

- Light sensitivity (1–10): ____

- Temperature sensitivity (1–10): ____

SECTION 4, EMOTIONAL SYSTEM AUDIT

Nighttime emotional load, stress, and trauma echoes.

4.1 Emotional Activation (1–10)

- anxiety before bed: ____

- anxiety during awakenings: ____

- rumination intensity: ____

- emotional flashbacks: ____

- fear of not sleeping: ____

- emotional loneliness at night: ____

4.2 Trauma & Hypervigilance Patterns (check all that apply)

☐ PTSD diagnosis
☐ trauma-linked dreams
☐ auditory sensitivity at night
☐ fear of silence
☐ sleeping with TV/noise for safety
☐ scanning the room
☐ sensitivity to footsteps/doors
☐ waking up in panic

4.3 Emotional Load of Daily Life

Check all that apply:
☐ relationship tension
☐ children's needs
☐ work pressure
☐ financial stress
☐ caregiving
☐ unresolved conflict
☐ grief

SECTION 5, COGNITIVE ACTIVATION AUDIT

The thought patterns that disrupt descent.

5.1 Thought Themes at Night (1–10)

Rate:

- problem-solving: ____
- mental rehearsing: ____
- catastrophizing: ____
- overthinking conversations: ____
- planning the next day: ____
- replaying past events: ____

5.2 Thought Style

Check any:
- ☐ fast-moving thoughts
- ☐ looping thoughts
- ☐ obsessive thinking
- ☐ worry-based thinking
- ☐ performance-based thinking
- ☐ existential or "big picture" thinking

SECTION 6, ENVIRONMENT & SENSORY AUDIT

6.1 Sensory Triggers (1–10)

Rate:

- noise sensitivity: ____
- light sensitivity: ____
- temperature disruptions: ____

- clutter-induced stress: ____

- sensory overstimulation in home: ____

6.2 Bedroom Dynamics

Check all:

☐ sleep space feels chaotic

☐ reminders of unfinished tasks

☐ emotionally charged objects

☐ partner snores/moves

☐ pets wake you

☐ shared bedtime conflicts

SECTION 7, LIFESTYLE & RELATIONAL AUDIT

7.1 Lifestyle Rhythm

Check:

☐ travel

☐ inconsistent schedule

☐ caregiving

☐ high-demand career

☐ late work hours

☐ unmanaged stress cycles

7.2 Social/Relational Activation

Rate (1–10):

- emotional support at home: ____

- household pace: ____

- relational tension affecting sleep: ____

- feeling "on call" for others: ____

SECTION 8, RECOVERY CAPACITY PROFILE

8.1 Recovery After Bad Nights (1–10)

Rate:

- ability to bounce back: ____

- tendency to spiral mentally: ____

- confidence in recovering: ____

- reliance on coping habits (screens/food/etc.): ____

- emotional resilience after poor sleep: ____

8.2 Personal Reset Skill

Rate:

- ability to identify misalignment quickly: ____

- ability to self-calm: ____

- belief in your body's ability to sleep: ____

SECTION 9, YOUR SLEEP PROFILE SUMMARY

Your personalized misalignment map.

Top Behavioral Misalignments

1. ____

2. ____

3. ____

Top Biological Misalignments

1. ____

2. ____

3. ____

Top Emotional Misalignments

1. ____

2. ____

3. ____

Top Cognitive Activators

1. ____

2. ____

Environmental Triggers

1. ____

2. ____

Primary Sleep Breakers

1. ____

2. ____

3. ____

Greatest Opportunities for Repair

1. ____

2. ____

3. ____

WHAT TO DO NEXT

After completing the audit:

1. Go to **Appendix B: Sleep Breakers Map** to visualize your patterns.

2. Then **Appendix C: The 7-Day Reset** to stabilize your systems.

3. Use **D–F** (Breathing, Evening Rituals, Morning Reset) to strengthen alignment.

4. Reassess after 7 days.

5. Watch your scores, and your nights, begin to shift.

This audit is your turning point.

APPENDIX B - THE SLEEP BREAKERS MAP

Your visual guide to understanding the root causes of your sleeplessness.

The Sleep Audit you just completed gave you **scores**.
The Sleep Breakers Map gives you **meaning**.

This appendix shows you how your:

- behaviors

- biology

- emotions

- thoughts

- environment

- lifestyle

…all connect to create the patterns you feel at night.

Your misalignments are not random.
They cluster.
They reinforce each other.
They follow predictable patterns.

The Sleep Breakers Map helps you see those patterns clearly, often for the first time in your life.

The Purpose of This Map

Most people try to fix sleep by attacking symptoms:

- "I can't fall asleep."

- "I wake up at 3 a.m."

- "I overthink at night."

- "I feel wired at bedtime."

But symptoms don't come out of nowhere.

They come from **sleep breakers**, the root drivers hidden underneath your experience.

This map shows you:

1. **Where your biggest misalignments are located**

2. **How those misalignments interact**

3. **Which system is creating the most nightly disruption**

4. **What needs to be addressed first**

5. **Your personal path to the fastest improvement**

Think of this map as the "MRI" of your sleep.

How the Map Works

There are **six core Breaker Zones**:

1. **Behavioral Breakers**

2. **Biological Breakers**

3. **Emotional Breakers**

4. **Cognitive Breakers**

5. **Environmental Breakers**

6. **Lifestyle Breakers**

Each zone contains **specific patterns** that you identified in Appendix A.

Your goal in this appendix:

Step 1: Identify which zones your highest scores fell into

Step 2: Note which zones cluster together

Step 3: Identify your "Primary Breaker Zone"

Step 4: Track the crossover effects (where one zone triggers another)

Step 5: Complete your Sleep Breaker Profile

When you finish this map, you'll know exactly why you struggle, and exactly what needs to change.

THE SIX BREAKER ZONES (Visual Map)

Think of it as a map you fill in mentally as you go.

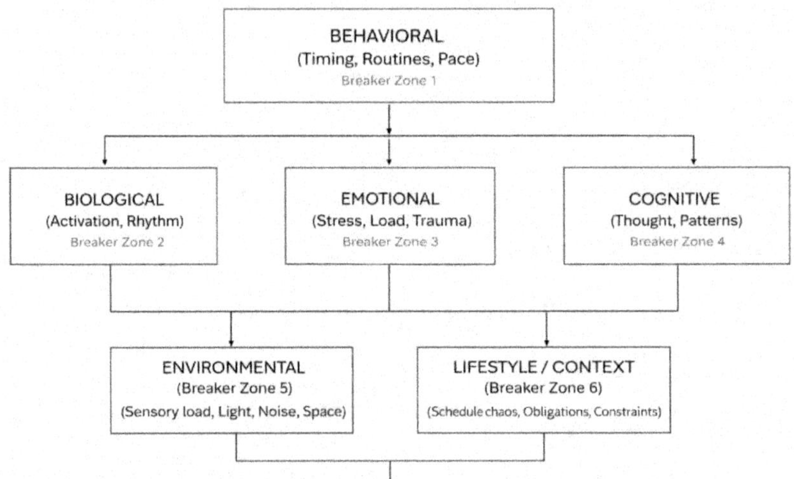

This model mirrors the reality of sleep:

Your nights are shaped by your days.
Your experience is shaped by your systems.
Your systems influence one another.

BREAKER ZONE 1, Behavioral Sleep Breakers (Section 2 from Audit)

If your Behavioral scores were highest… start here.

These include:

- inconsistent bed/wake times

- chaotic evenings

- late eating

- late work

- overstimulation

- no wind-down

- pushing past tiredness

- multitasking at night

Behavioral → Biological Crossover

Behavioral misalignment almost always triggers:

- physiological activation

- "second wind"

- unstable circadian rhythm

Behavioral → Emotional Crossover

Leads to:

- nighttime anxiety

- feeling "behind"

- emotional overflow at night

If this zone is your highest, **your nights break because your *patterns* break.**

BREAKER ZONE 2, Biological Sleep Breakers (Section 3 from Audit)

If your Biological scores were highest… this is your foundation.

Includes:

- tension

- overheating

- heart rate spikes

- circadian confusion

- caffeine/alcohol sensitivity

- restlessness

Common triggers

- stress physiology

- overdrive lifestyle

- hormonal misalignment

- poor light environment

Biological → Cognitive Crossover

When biology spikes, the mind often follows:

- racing thoughts

- hyperfocus

- "wired but tired" states

Biological → Emotional Crossover

Leads to:

- irrational worry

- nighttime dread

- emotional volatility

If this is your strongest zone, **your nights break because your *body* stays in overdrive.**

BREAKER ZONE 3, Emotional Sleep Breakers (Section 4 from Audit)

This is one of the most overlooked, and most powerful, zones.

Includes:

- nighttime anxiety

- emotional memories

- fear of night

- fear of waking

- PTSD patterns

- hypervigilance

- emotional loneliness

Emotional → Biological Crossover

Triggers:

- activation

- heart rate spikes

- breathing changes

- muscle tension

Emotional → Cognitive Crossover

Triggers:

- rumination

- catastrophizing

- mental spirals

If this zone is dominant, your nights break because your **emotions become louder than your environment**.

BREAKER ZONE 4, Cognitive Sleep Breakers (Section 5 from Audit)

If your thoughts dominate your nights…

Includes:

- planning

- replaying

- analyzing

- problem-solving

- rehearsing

- catastrophizing

- existential thoughts

Cognitive → Emotional Crossover

Thoughts create:

- anxiety

- dread

- guilt

- worry

Cognitive → Behavioral Crossover

Leads to:

- avoiding bedtime

- delaying wind-down

- needing distraction

If this is your zone, your nights break because your **<u>mind won't stop talking</u>**.

BREAKER ZONE 5, Environmental Sleep Breakers (Section 6 from Audit)

Includes:

- noise

- light

- clutter

- uncomfortable bed

- partner disruptions

- emotional tension in the home

If this zone was high, your nights break because your **environment keeps your systems activated**.

BREAKER ZONE 6, Lifestyle Sleep Breakers (Section 7 from Audit)

Includes:

- high-performance lifestyle

- travel

- irregular schedules

- overcommitment

- emotional caregiving

- constant pressure

If this zone is high, your nights break because **your life has no "off switch."**

HOW TO CREATE YOUR SLEEP BREAKER PROFILE

Step 1, List your top 3–5 highest scores from Appendix A

(Behavioral, Biological, Emotional, Cognitive, Environmental, Lifestyle)

Step 2, Place each one into the correct Breaker Zone

Example:

- racing thoughts → Cognitive

- heart rate spikes → Biological

- inconsistent bedtime → Behavioral

Step 3, Identify your Primary Breaker Zone

This is the zone with the highest scores.

Step 4, Identify your Secondary Zones

The two zones that feed into your primary misalignment.

Step 5, Name your Sleep Breaker Pattern

Here are the six most common:

1. **The Wired Performer**
   (high Biological + high Lifestyle)

2. **The Emotional Keeper**
   (high Emotional + high Cognitive)

3. **The Rhythm Disruptor**
   (high Behavioral + high Biological)

4. **The Hypervigilant Sleeper**
   (high Emotional + high Environmental)

5. **The Chaotic Cycler**
    (high Behavioral + high Lifestyle)

6. **The Suppressed Descender**
    (high Cognitive + high Biological)

Step 6, Write your final Sleep Breaker Profile statement

Example:

"My Primary Breaker Zone is Biological, supported by Emotional misalignment. My sleep breaks because my body stays activated at night, which triggers emotional spikes and cognitive loops."

This statement becomes the core of your 7-Day Reset.

NEXT STEP

Your Sleep Breaker Profile tells you exactly **why** you struggle.

Now turn to:

Appendix C, The 7-Day Reset

This is where you begin stabilizing your systems and rebuilding predictable, peaceful nights.

APPENDIX C - THE 7-DAY RESET

A guided, step-by-step realignment of your Behavioral, Biological, and Emotional systems.

This is the Dreameaz foundational reset.

It's not a detox.
It's not a fast.
It's not a challenge or bootcamp.
There is no extremity here.

This is a **systemic recalibration**, a way to restore predictability to your nights by stabilizing the systems that carry you through the day.

You are not fixing sleep directly.
You are restoring the *conditions* that allow sleep to return on its own.

In seven days, you won't become a perfect sleeper,
but you **will** feel your body shift back toward alignment.

You will feel:

- calmer evenings

- reduced nighttime activation

- earlier natural sleep pressure

- fewer spirals

- morning clarity

- emotional softness

- biological predictability

- confidence

- safety in your own rhythms

This is the turning point.

HOW THE RESET WORKS

The 7-Day Reset focuses on three pillars:

1. Stabilize the Behavioral System

Create structure, rhythm, predictability.

2. Soothe the Biological System

Reduce activation, restore the body's sleep slope.

3. Ground the Emotional System

Prevent nighttime emotional load from spilling into the dark.

Each day includes:

- one **behavioral anchor**
- one **biological soothe**
- one **emotional grounding practice**
- one **evening wind-down adjustment**
- one **morning reset ritual**
- and one **nighttime protocol** for if you wake up

This is the light version.
The full extended version, the 21-Day Deep Reset, is part of the Dreameaz Course.

But this 7-day version is enough to create real movement in your sleep.

IMPORTANT BEFORE STARTING

You do **not** need perfect days.
You do **not** need to eliminate stress.
You do **not** need to change your entire life.

Your goal for 7 days is simple:

Follow the alignment actions.
Don't judge your nights.
Let your systems settle.

Sleep improves naturally when your systems stop fighting each other.

THE 7-DAY RESET

DAY 1, Stabilize the Ground

Goal: Begin reducing chaos and unpredictability.

Behavioral Anchor

Set a *fixed wake time* for all 7 days.
No exceptions, no changes, no snoozing.

Biological Soothe

Hydrate early; stop caffeine after 1 p.m.

Emotional Grounding

10 minutes of quiet reflection or journaling:

- What are you carrying?

- What needs to be released today?

Evening Adjustment

Turn off bright overhead lighting 1 hour before bed.
Use soft, warm light only.

Morning Reset

5 minutes of natural light within an hour of waking.

DAY 2, Lower the Body's Alarm

Goal: Reduce baseline physiological activation.

Behavioral Anchor

No work, planning, or problem-solving 60 minutes before bed.

Biological Soothe

10 slow nose breaths (inhale 4 seconds, exhale 6 seconds) at three points:

- mid-day

- late afternoon

- pre-bed

Emotional Grounding

Write down:

- What you fear about sleep

- What is actually true
  This separates emotion from reality.

Evening Adjustment

Cool the bedroom to 65–68°F.

Morning Reset

2 minutes of cold water on wrists/face for cortisol grounding.

DAY 3, Quiet the Mind's Loops

Goal: Reduce mental spiraling and cognitive overactivation.

Behavioral Anchor

A 15-minute "mental download" before evening:

- open tasks

- decisions

- worries

- tomorrow's steps

This prevents nighttime rumination.

Biological Soothe

Gentle stretching for 5–7 minutes before bed:

- neck

- shoulders

- hips

- lower back

Emotional Grounding

The 4-sentence release:

1. "I can let today be over."

2. "My body knows how to rest."

3. "I am allowed to feel supported."

4. "The night is safe for me."

Evening Adjustment

Screens off 45 minutes before bed.

Morning Reset

Walk for 5 minutes outdoors.

DAY 4, Rebuild the Clock

Goal: Strengthen circadian consistency.

Behavioral Anchor

Eat all meals within a 12-hour window.

Biological Soothe

Light exposure:

- bright morning light
- dim evening light

Emotional Grounding

Name the emotional weight you're holding.
Tell your body: "We won't solve this at night."

Evening Adjustment

Same wind-down start time as Day 3.

Morning Reset

Deep breathing + sunlight + steady movement (2–3 minutes each).

DAY 5, Release Stored Tension

Goal: Reduce accumulated stress load.

Behavioral Anchor

No emotional conversations after 8 p.m.

Biological Soothe

Warm shower or bath 60–90 minutes before bed to trigger post-cooling.

Emotional Grounding

3-minute "safe place visualization":
Imagine a place where nothing is demanded of you.

Evening Adjustment

Place your phone across the room or outside the bedroom.

Morning Reset

Drink water promptly upon waking.

DAY 6, Calm the Emotional Echo

Goal: Reduce nighttime emotional activation.

Behavioral Anchor

A 15-minute buffer between your final activity and the start of your wind-down.

Biological Soothe

Slow exhale breathing before bed (inhale 3, exhale 7).

Emotional Grounding

Ask yourself:
"What emotion am I carrying that doesn't belong in the dark?"

Release it intentionally.

Evening Adjustment

No TV in bed or falling asleep to screens.

Morning Reset

10 deep breaths + exposure to morning noise (birds, outside sounds).

DAY 7, Reinforce the Descent

Goal: Integrate all three systems into a predictable bedtime descent.

Behavioral Anchor

Keep the same bedtime window (within 30 minutes).

Biological Soothe

Light stretching + warm drink (herbal tea).

Emotional Grounding

A 2-minute gratitude reflection:

- what went right today

- what softened

- what surprised you

Evening Adjustment

Darken the room fully.
Use blackout if needed.

Morning Reset

Repeat the same morning routine as Day 6.

THE NIGHTTIME PROTOCOL (used every night of the reset)

If you wake up:

1. Stay still for 10–15 seconds

Let the body calm before the mind activates.

2. Ask: "Is this biological, emotional, or cognitive?"

One question brings awareness and removes panic.

3. Breathe slowly through the nose

Inhale 4 seconds → Exhale 8 seconds.

4. Repeat the grounding phrase:

"I am safe. My body knows how to return."

5. If still awake after ~20 minutes:

Sit up, dim light only, and do one quiet activity:

- slow reading

- soft stretching

- light journaling

Return to bed when your body softens, not before.

WHAT TO EXPECT BY DAY 7

You will likely feel:

- calmer nights

- fewer spikes

- more predictable sleepiness

- reduced rumination

- emotional stability

- earlier descent into rest

- morning clarity

- confidence returning

Your nights may not be perfect,
but your *systems* will feel steadier.

That is the win.

The reset doesn't fix sleep.
It fixes the **conditions** that let sleep return.

WHAT HAPPENS AFTER DAY 7

At the end of Day 7:

- Revisit Appendix A

- Rescore your highest scores

- Notice what changed

- Identify new misalignments

- Then continue implementing the elements that helped most

If you want deeper transformation and personalization, the full Dreameaz 21-Day Reset and expanded assessment are available at dreameaz.com.

How to calm your body, quiet your mind, and guide yourself into descent.

Breathing is the bridge between your body and your mind.
It is the only system you can control from both directions:

- When your **mind** is overstimulated, breath brings it down.

- When your **body** is activated, breath slows it.

- When your **emotions** are overloaded, breath grounds them.

Most people underestimate the role of breathing in sleep because they've never experienced what it feels like to truly shift their physiology.

This appendix teaches you the Dreameaz breathing practices designed specifically for sleep descent, emotional grounding, panic interruption, and nighttime awakenings.

These practices are:

- simple

- safe

- natural

- fast

- and aligned with the nervous system

You don't need experience.
You don't need training.
You only need a few quiet minutes.

WHY BREATHING MATTERS FOR SLEEP

Your nights depend on your nervous system.
Your nervous system depends on your breath.

When you breathe:

- **fast**, your body believes it's in danger.

- **slow**, your body believes it's safe.

- **shallow**, your mind stays on edge.

- **deep**, your body shifts toward descent.

Your breath is your internal signal system.

It tells your body:

- "It's time to fight."

- "It's time to work."

- "It's time to think."

- "It's time to rest."

This section gives you the exact tools to send the message your body has been waiting for:

"You can let go now."

THE FOUR CORE DREAMEAZ BREATHING PRACTICES

Each practice serves a different function:

1. **The Descent Breath** – for falling asleep

2. **The Nervous System Reset Breath** – for biological overactivation

3. **The Emotional Softening Breath** – for fear, loneliness, and heaviness

4. **The 3AM Rescue Breath** – for nighttime awakenings

You can use these anytime, anywhere, without needing a yoga mat, a quiet room, or a perfect setup.

Let's begin.

1. THE DESCENT BREATH

For falling asleep and easing into your wind-down.

This breath is designed to:

- flatten your stress curve

- lower your heart rate

- soften muscle tension

- prepare your body for sleep pressure

It is the simplest but most powerful practice.

How to Do It

1. Inhale through your nose for **4 seconds**.

2. Exhale through your nose for **6 seconds**.

3. Repeat gently for **3–5 minutes**.

Why It Works

The longer exhale does two things:

- activates the parasympathetic nervous system

- signals "safety" to your brainstem

Your brainstem controls sleep.
You are speaking directly to it.

When to Use It

- before bed

- during your wind-down

- while reading or relaxing

- after a stressful evening

This breath is the "off switch" most people don't know they have.

2. THE NERVOUS SYSTEM RESET BREATH

For calming overactivation and physiological spikes.

This is for:

- heart racing

- tension

- overheating

- adrenaline surges

- chest tightness

- restlessness

How to Do It

1. Inhale through your nose for **3 seconds**.

2. Hold for **1 second**.

3. Exhale through pursed lips for **7 seconds**.

Do this 6–10 times.

Why It Works

The pursed-lip exhale creates **back pressure** in the lungs, slowing heart rate almost instantly.
The short inhale prevents over breathing.
The long exhale dampens adrenaline.

This is the fastest way to neutralize your fight-or-flight system without medication or white-knuckle effort.

When to Use It

- after evening stress

- when your day feels too heavy

- when your heart won't slow down

- when your body feels "wired but tired"

- before beginning your wind-down

- anytime you feel physiological overdrive

This breath resets the biological system.

3. THE EMOTIONAL SOFTENING BREATH

For emotional heaviness, sadness, trauma echoes, and nighttime vulnerability.

Nighttime can pull emotions to the surface.
This breath creates softness where the body has braced.

How to Do It

1. Inhale gently for **4 seconds**.

2. Exhale with an audible sigh for **8 seconds**.

3. Let your shoulders fall as you exhale.

4. Repeat 5–8 times.

Why It Works

The sigh releases:

- held emotional tension

- stored sadness

- internal bracing

- the "I must stay in control" feeling

It also triggers oxytocin release, the hormone of comfort, safety, and connection.

When to Use It

- before bed if you feel emotional

- after an argument

- when loneliness rises

- when fear of the night appears

- when memories feel loud

- when grief hits unexpectedly

This breath tells your heart: **"You're safe now."**

4. THE 3AM RESCUE BREATH

For nighttime awakenings, panic waves, or alertness spikes.

If you wake up with:

- panic

- confusion

- adrenaline

- heart rate spikes

- emotional echoes

- racing thoughts

This is your rescue breath.

How to Do It

1. Inhale **through the nose** for **4 seconds**.

2. Hold for **2 seconds**.

3. Exhale **through the mouth** for **8 seconds**.

4. Repeat for **2–4 minutes**.

Why It Works

Nighttime awakenings often trigger:

- cortisol elevation

- adrenaline release

- hypervigilance

The hold at the top signals control and stabilization.
The extended exhale counters the adrenaline rush.
The mouth exhale releases emotional tension.

When to Use It

- any nighttime awakening

- any 3AM spiral

- after a nightmare

- after a sudden panic jolt

- when you feel "stuck awake"

This practice often shortens awakenings dramatically.

THE BREATHING TRIAD: A SIMPLE SUMMARY

If you want the simplest formula:

- **Long exhale = calm body**

- **Gentle inhale = calm mind**

- **Sigh = calm emotions**

That's the entire nervous system in three breaths.

HOW TO USE THESE PRACTICES IN YOUR NIGHTLY ROUTINE

Before Bed

Choose one:

- Descent Breath

- Emotional Softening Breath

During Stressful Evenings

Use:

- Nervous System Reset Breath

During Awakenings

Always use:

- 3AM Rescue Breath

During High-Performance Days

Use:

- Reset Breath midday

- Descent Breath evening

After Conflict or Emotional Load

Use:

- Emotional Softening Breath

You do not need to master everything.
Use what your body responds to.
Use what softens you fastest.
Use what makes you feel safe.

WHEN TO STOP A PRACTICE

Stop when:

- your breath feels automatic

- your body loosens

- your thoughts slow

- your chest softens

- your shoulders drop

- you feel warmth or a wave of calm

That means your system has shifted.

CLOSING NOTE

Breathing is not a magic trick.
It's a physiological mechanism that tells your body the truth:

**"You can stop fighting.
You can let go.
You can descend."**

Every night of your life… your breath can guide you home.

APPENDIX E - EVENING RITUAL TEMPLATES

Predictable wind-downs that restore alignment and guide your body toward sleep.

Most people think rituals are about discipline.

They're not.

Rituals are about *signals*, clear, consistent cues that tell your Behavioral System to slow down, your Biological System to descend, and your Emotional System to soften.

These templates are not rules.
They're invitations.

Use them as written, blend them, or customize them.
Over time, your body will learn: **"This is when we let go."**

A Note Before You Begin

These are the **core templates** from the Dreameaz model, the ones designed specifically for book readers.

If you want the full suite of templates (10+ evening rituals including ones for shift workers, parents, chaos evenings, trauma-informed cycles, performance seasons, and insomnia-specific routines), they are available anytime at:

dreameaz.com

But for now, the templates below will give you everything you need to begin transforming your nights.

EVENING RITUAL TEMPLATE #1

1. The Fast 15-Minute Reset Ritual

For the nights when you're tired, busy, or overwhelmed.

This is the ritual you use when life is messy and you don't have time for anything elaborate.
It's short, effective, and hits all three systems.

Minute 0–3, Environmental Shift

- turn off overhead lights

- switch to warm lighting

- silence notifications

- place your phone out of arm's reach

This reduces Behavioral chaos and Biological stimulation.

Minute 3–7, Breath & Body

Choose *one*:

- 3 minutes of Descent Breath

- or 2 minutes of gentle neck/shoulder stretching

- or 90 seconds of slow exhale breathing

This calms your nervous system quickly.

Minute 7–12, Emotional Lightening

Write down:

- one thing you're carrying

- one thing you're releasing

Then whisper:
"The day is finished."

Minute 12–15, Descent Cue

Do one soft, predictable action:

- wash your face

- dim your room

- pour herbal tea

- change into sleep clothing

This anchors your system.
Your body recognizes the sequence.

Use this ritual on chaotic nights.
It's fast, but extremely effective.

EVENING RITUAL TEMPLATE #2

2. The Standard 60-Minute Dreameaz Wind-Down

The signature ritual for deep, predictable descent.

This ritual matches the structure used in Chapter 12 and the Dreameaz method.

Minute 0–10, Release the Day

- lights down

- screens off

- room temperature lowered

- do a brief 2–3 minute breath

- say out loud: "The day is done."

This closes the Behavioral System.

Minute 10–25, Biological Softening

Choose one:

- warm shower

- full-body stretching

- slow walking around the home

- self-massage (neck, jaw, temples)

This reduces physical activation.

Minute 25–40, Emotional Grounding

Options:

- journal for 10 minutes

- gratitude reflection

- safe place visualization

- quiet music or calming soundscape

This drains emotional residue from the day.

Minute 40–55, Gentle Descent

- dim or turn off lights

- use a bedside lamp only

- read something light or comforting

- slow breathing

Minute 55–60, Final Cue

- enter your bed slowly

- arrange pillows

- one final long exhale

- "My body knows the way down."

This is the ideal nightly ritual for most readers.

EVENING RITUAL TEMPLATE #3

3. The Trauma-Safe Wind-Down

For nights with emotional echoes, hypervigilance, or PTSD patterns.

Nighttime can feel vulnerable when the nervous system is carrying old experiences.
This ritual is built for safety, softness, and grounding.

Minute 0–5, Establish Safety

- turn on soft lighting

- close the blinds

- check the home (once only)

- create a settled environment

Repeat softly:
"I am safe in this space."

Minute 5–15, Breath for the Heart

Use the **Emotional Softening Breath** (inhale 4, sigh out 8).

If emotions rise, let them.

Minute 15–25, Weighted Grounding

Use one:

- weighted blanket

- heavy comforter

- warm compress on chest or abdomen

- hand over heart + slow breathing

This signals safety to your vagus nerve.

Minute 25–40, Emotional Release Option

Choose what feels right:

- journaling

- drawing

- crying

- listening to calming music

- holding something comforting (blanket, pillow, object)

No judgment.
No analysis.
Just release.

Minute 40–50, Sensory Soothing

- lavender or soft essential oil

- gentle stretching

- light touch over arms/shoulders

- warm drink

Minute 50–55, Bedtime Reinforcement

Whisper:
"Nothing is being asked of me right now."

This ritual turns fear into softness.

4. The High-Performance Decompression Ritual

For overachievers, intense professionals, or anyone who stays "on" all day.

If your mind is sharp, driven, and always working, you don't need peace, you need *decompression*.

Minute 0–10, Cognitive Offload

Write down:

- unresolved tasks

- decisions waiting on you

- pressure you're carrying

This moves mental load *out* of your head.

Minute 10–20, Biological Discharge

Your body has stored adrenaline.
Remove it with:

- a 10-minute walk

- light cycling

- simple mobility

Not exercise, just movement.

Minute 20–35, Nervous System Reset

Use the **Reset Breath** (inhale 3, hold 1, exhale 7).
This stops the "second wind."

Minute 35–45, Mental Narrowing

Do one simple, low-cognitive activity:

- folding clothes

- light cleaning

- organizing your nightstand

- stretching

Choose something that narrows mental focus without stimulating.

Minute 45–60, Transition to Bed

- dim light

- soft music

- shut down all digital interfaces

- warm shower

- enter bed slowly

This ritual turns intensity into calm.

5. The Emotional Release Ritual

For nights when your heart is heavier than your body.

This ritual helps when you feel:

- sadness

- loneliness

- grief

- overwhelm

- emotional residue

- relationship tension

Minute 0–10, Emotional Honesty Moment

Sit in low light.
Ask yourself:
"What am I truly feeling?"

Name it.
Don't fix it.

Minute 10–20, Emotional Softening Breath

Use sighing exhalations.
Let your shoulders fall.

Minute 20–35, Gentle Expression

Choose one:

- write a letter you won't send

- journal freely

- cry

- draw

- doodle

- talk softly to yourself

- hold a comforting item

This releases pressure from the emotional system.

Minute 35–45, Comfort Cue

- warm tea

- soft blanket

- warm compress

- quiet music

Minute 45–60, Return to Safety

Whisper internally:
"This emotion can exist without taking my night."

This ritual prevents emotional overflow at bedtime.

6. The Minimalist Ritual (For People Who "Don't Do Rituals")

Simple. Quick. Effective.

If structure stresses you out…
or if you hate routines…
or if you get overwhelmed by too many steps…

This ritual is for you.

3 Simple Steps

Step 1: Dim the Environment (3–5 minutes)

- lights down

- sound lowered

- screens off

- slow pacing

Step 2: Calm the Body (3–5 minutes)

Choose one:

- 5 slow breaths

- 5 gentle stretches

- warm face rinse

- soft music

Step 3: Cue the Descent (1 minute)

Do one predictable cue:

- get into bed

- pull covers up

- take one long exhale

That's it.
No complexity.
No resistance.

Less is often more.

FINAL NOTE

Your evening ritual is not about perfection.
It's about repetition.

When your body sees the same signals night after night, it begins to anticipate sleep rather than fear it.

That anticipation is descent.
Descent is alignment.
Alignment is rest.

Your nights change when your evenings become predictable.

APPENDIX F - MORNING RESET GUIDE

How to anchor your days, stabilize your biology, and protect your nights.

Sleep does not begin at night.

It begins in the **first 60 minutes of your morning**.

What you do upon waking determines:

- your cortisol rhythm

- your alertness curve

- your emotional load

- your stress slope

- your biological safety signals

- your nighttime descent

Most people sabotage their sleep before they finish their first cup of coffee.

This guide shows you how to build mornings that support you, even during chaos, high-pressure seasons, or emotionally heavy times.

The Morning Reset is not about productivity.
It's not about discipline.
It's not about doing more.

It's about **creating the internal conditions that make restful nights possible.**

A Note Before You Begin

This Morning Reset Guide is the **core version**, built for book readers.

The full extended Morning Reset Protocol, including performance-specific routines, PTSD-adjusted morning activations, anxiety-calming morning cycles, and full circadian coaching, is available at:

dreameaz.com

This guide gives you everything you need to begin.

WHY MORNINGS MATTER FOR SLEEP

Your morning shapes:

- cortisol

- alertness rhythms

- circadian timing

- energy waves

- emotional resilience

- nighttime calm

A chaotic morning leads to:

- unpredictable evenings

- irregular sleep pressure

- nighttime alertness

- trouble falling asleep

- 3AM awakenings

A grounded morning leads to:

- steady energy

- calmer emotional baseline

- smoother descent at night

- consistent sleep drive

- less rumination

- fewer awakenings

A morning reset is not optional.
It's foundational.

THE SIX FOUNDATIONAL MORNING RESET ELEMENTS

You don't need to do all of them every day.
You simply need *some* of them, consistently.

Below are the six elements your system needs most:

1. **Light Exposure**

2. **Movement**

3. **Breath**

4. **Hydration**

5. **Emotional Orientation**

6. **Task Simplification**

Let's break them down.

1. LIGHT EXPOSURE

The single most powerful circadian anchor.

Within 60 minutes of waking:

- go outside

- open blinds

- face windows

- get direct or indirect sunlight

2–10 minutes is enough.

If sunlight is unavailable:

- use indoor bright light

- stand near a window

- turn on strong room lighting

Why it works:
Light hits photoreceptors → signals the brain → regulates cortisol → sets your 24-hour clock → determines nighttime sleepiness.

More morning light = deeper nighttime descent.

2. MOVEMENT

The body must wake for the mind to calm.

Movement doesn't mean exercise.

Movement means:

- walking around your kitchen

- stretching spine/hips

- shaking out arms

- gentle mobility

- a slow walk outside

2–5 minutes changes your biological baseline.

Movement clears overnight stagnation and signals:
"The day has begun."

That signal matters.

3. BREATH

Resetting the nervous system before stress sets in.

Use one of these each morning:

- 10 slow breaths (inhale 4, exhale 6)

- 1 minute of deep nose breathing

- 5 slow sighs (inhale 4, sigh out 8)

- the Reset Breath (inhale 3, hold 1, exhale 7)

Morning breathwork:

- reduces anxiety spikes

- stabilizes emotions

- lowers cortisol reactivity

- improves clarity

This is your emotional anchor.

4. HYDRATION

Water before caffeine.

Before your first caffeine hit:

- drink a glass of water

- add electrolytes if needed

- sip slowly

This:

- wakes digestion

- grounds cortisol

- supports mood regulation

- reduces afternoon crashes

Caffeine without water = biological chaos.

5. EMOTIONAL ORIENTATION

Set the tone before the world takes it from you.

Take **2 minutes** to ask:

- "What do I need today?"

- "What is eating at me?"

- "What can wait?"

Choose one grounding practice:

- gratitude for 60 seconds

- brief journaling

- a calming affirmation

- a soft thought ("I don't have to carry everything at once.")

- intentional stillness

This stabilizes your Emotional System early.

It is harder for anxiety to hijack your night when the morning is emotionally clear.

6. TASK SIMPLIFICATION

Your brain needs clarity, not chaos.

Spend **less than 2 minutes** doing this:

- write down the top 3 priorities of the day

- everything else gets categorized as:

o   "Later"

o   "Optional"

o   "Not today"

This stops cognitive overload, the type that spills into your nights.

FOUR MORNING RESET ROUTINES

Below are four templates you can use anytime.

MORNING RESET TEMPLATE #1

1. The 5-Minute Alignment Reset

For chaotic mornings or limited time.

Minute 0–1
Open blinds or step outside.

Minute 1–2
Drink a glass of water.

Minute 2–3
Take 5 slow breaths.

Minute 3–5
Do light stretching or walk around your home.

Done.
Your body is anchored.

MORNING RESET TEMPLATE #2

2. The 15-Minute Calm & Clear Routine

For grounding anxiety and stabilizing emotions.

Minute 0–2
Light exposure.

Minute 2–4
Hydration.

Minute 4–7
Reset Breath (inhale 3, hold 1, exhale 7).

Minute 7–10
Gentle movement.

Minute 10–15
Emotional orientation or journaling.

This is the best routine for high-stress seasons.

MORNING RESET TEMPLATE #3

3. The High-Performance Activation Routine

For professionals, entrepreneurs, and intense workloads.

Minute 0–3
High-intensity light exposure.

Minute 3–5
Movement with intention:

- brisk walk

- short mobility flow

Minute 5–8
Reset Breath.

Minute 8–10
Set the "Top 3 Tasks."

Minute 10–15
Light breakfast or protein.

This increases cognitive readiness while preventing burnout cycles.

MORNING RESET TEMPLATE #4

4. The Emotional Safety Morning (PTSD-Friendly)

For people with trauma echoes, nighttime fear, or emotional vulnerability.

Minute 0–2
Slow, soft light. No abrupt brightness.

Minute 2–4
Warm water or tea.

Minute 4–7
Emotional Softening Breath (sigh out).

Minute 7–10
Weighted grounding or holding something comforting.

Minute 10–12
Repeat: "Nothing is demanded of me right now."

This routine establishes safety before activation.

THE MORNING RESET RULES

Keep it simple.
Keep it predictable.
Keep it gentle.

Rule #1: Never skip light.

Even on bad nights.

Rule #2: Never start the day with your phone.

You lose your emotional footing instantly.

Rule #3: One minute is better than none.

There is no perfect morning.

Rule #4: Emotional clarity is more important than productivity.

A calm morning protects your night.

Rule #5: Consistency beats intensity.

Small, steady wins realign your system.

WHAT TO EXPECT AFTER A WEEK OF MORNING RESETS

Most people report:

- smoother energy

- calmer evenings

- fewer spirals at bedtime

- earlier natural sleepiness

- reduced nighttime anxiety

- fewer 3AM awakenings

- emotional steadiness

- a feeling of "more space" in the mind

Morning resets create long-term stability.
They are your daily alignment anchor.

Your nights return when your mornings lead.

APPENDIX G, TOOLS & RESOURCES

Everything you need to support alignment, stabilize your systems, and build long-term sleep resilience.

Restful sleep isn't created by a single habit.
It's built through an environment, a rhythm, a set of tools, and gentle supports that help your mind, body, and emotions realign, even during stress, trauma echoes, performance cycles, or chaotic seasons.

This appendix gathers the most helpful, research-backed, real-world tools that complement the Dreameaz method.
They are practical, accessible, and designed to help you soften your nights and protect your days.

Some tools you can begin using immediately.
Some are optional.
All are supportive.

BREATHING & NERVOUS SYSTEM SUPPORT

Descent Breath Audio

Guides you into relaxation through extended exhalation.

3AM Rescue Breath Audio

For calming awakenings and breaking the panic cycle.

Nervous System Reset Breath

A rapid biological downshift for evenings with overstimulation.

Emotional Softening Breath

Releases emotional load and restores safety.

SOUND & ENVIRONMENT SUPPORT

Sleep Noise Tracks

- white noise
- pink noise
- brown noise
- low-frequency hums

Nature Sounds

- rainfall
- ocean waves
- running water
- wind through trees

Environmental Tools

- warm lighting
- bedside dimmers
- blackout solutions
- cooling bedding
- breathable sleepwear

CBT & COGNITIVE SUPPORT

Thought Download Template

A simple structure for reducing nighttime cognitive load.

3AM Cognitive Release Sheet

Stops rumination loops during awakenings.

Reframing Prompts

For fear of not sleeping, performance anxiety, or "what if" loops.

Identity Shift Scripts

To help rewrite your internal sleep story.

EMOTIONAL & TRAUMA-SAFE SUPPORT

Trauma-Safe Grounding Exercises

Gentle, body-based tools for hypervigilance.

Safe Place Visualization

A quick emotional anchor for difficult nights.

Nighttime Fear Release Prompts

For evenings carrying emotional weight.

Weighted Grounding Guidance

Using pressure for comfort without overheating.

BIOLOGICAL SUPPORT TOOLS

Circadian Light Tools

- sunrise lamps
- morning light protocols
- evening light filters

Temperature Regulation

- cooling pillows
- breathable bedding

- room temperature guide

Caffeine & Alcohol Timing Guides

Understand how timing impacts sleep pressure and nighttime stability.

Movement Timing Map

Shows when activity supports sleep, and when it sabotages it.

BEHAVIORAL SUPPORT TOOLS

Wind-Down Time Planner

A simple guide to anchor your nightly descent window.

Evening Simplification Checklist

Reduces decision fatigue before bed.

Predictable Sequence Builder

Helps you create a consistent pre-sleep rhythm.

In-Bed Behavior Guide

What to do (and what not to do) when lying awake.

MORNING RESET SUPPORT

Light Exposure Checklist

For stabilizing the circadian clock.

Mini Movement Routines

2–5 minute options for activating the body safely.

Hydration Formula

Supports cortisol regulation and morning clarity.

Top 3 Task Template

Prevents cognitive overload from bleeding into the night.

HIGH-PERFORMANCE RESOURCES

Cortisol Curve Tracker

Maps alertness and energy spikes across the day.

Screen & Meeting Timing Guide

Helps prevent evening overstimulation.

Stress Load Map

Identifies when daily emotional residue will affect sleep.

High-Performance Wind-Down Routines

Made for executives, entrepreneurs, and intense workloads.

RELATIONSHIP & HOME ENVIRONMENT SUPPORT

Partner Sleep Harmony Guide

For couples with different rhythms.

Co-Sleeping Map for Parents

Helps families stabilize evenings together.

Evening Home-Pace Guide

Moves the household toward calm instead of chaos.

Sleep-Safe Bedroom Design

How to build a room that cues descent and stability.

WHERE TO FIND ALL THESE TOOLS

Every tool listed in this appendix was designed to support the same alignment you've learned throughout this book, Behavioral, Biological, and Emotional.

Many readers use what's here and do incredibly well.
Others want deeper structure, audio guidance, full ritual libraries, or personalized support.

If you ever want the complete set of Dreameaz tools, you can find them anytime at:

Dreameaz.com

There you'll gain access to:

- the full **Dreameaz Comprehensive Sleep Diagnostic**

- the **21-Day Deep Reset Program**

- the entire **Breathing & Grounding Audio Library**

- expanded **PTSD-safe night practices**

- advanced **High-Performance Sleep Protocols**

- customizable **Evening & Morning Routine Builders**

- downloadable templates, maps, and guides

- curated sleep sounds and nature soundscapes

None of these are required.
They exist simply to support you as deeply as you choose to go.

Your transformation doesn't end with this book.
You now have a toolkit, and a home for your ongoing sleep journey whenever you need it.

REFERENCES

American Academy of Sleep Medicine. (2014). *International Classification of Sleep Disorders* (3rd ed.). Darien, IL: AASM.

Barbey, A. K. (2018). Network neuroscience theory of human intelligence. *Trends in Cognitive Sciences*, 22(1), 8–20.

Borbely, A. A. (1982). A two-process model of sleep regulation. *Human Neurobiology*, 1, 195–204.

Bowers, M. E., & Yehuda, R. (2016). Intergenerational transmission of stress in humans. *Neuropsychopharmacology*, 41, 232–244.

Buysse, D. J. (2014). Sleep health: Can we define it? Does it matter? *Sleep*, 37(1), 9–17.

Carskadon, M. A., & Dement, W. C. (2017). Sleep states and cycles. In M. Kryger, T. Roth, & W. C. Dement (Eds.), *Principles and Practice of Sleep Medicine* (6th ed.). Philadelphia: Elsevier.

Chrousos, G. P. (2009). Stress and disorders of the stress system. *Nature Reviews Endocrinology*, 5, 374–381.

Craig, A. D. (2009). How do you feel, now? The anterior insula and human awareness. *Nature Reviews Neuroscience*, 10, 59–70.

Davidson, R. J., & McEwen, B. S. (2012). Social influences on neuroplasticity: Stress and interventions to promote well-being. *Nature Neuroscience*, 15, 689–695.

Dinges, D. F. (1995). An overview of sleepiness and accidents. *Journal of Sleep Research*, 4(s2), 4–14.

Duhigg, C. (2012). *The Power of Habit*. New York: Random House.

Feldman, R. (2017). The neurobiology of human attachments. *Trends in Cognitive Sciences*, 21(2), 80–99.

Foster, R. G., & Kreitzman, L. (2014). *The Rhythms of Life: The Biological Clocks that Control the Daily Lives of Every Living Thing*. Yale University Press.

Goldstein, A. N., & Walker, M. P. (2014). The role of sleep in emotional brain regulation. *Annual Review of Clinical Psychology*, 10, 679–708.

Grandner, M. A. (2017). Sleep, health, and society. *Sleep Medicine Clinics*, 12, 1–22.

Harley, R. (2020). Nighttime physiology and emotional memory. *Journal of Neuroscience*, 40(2), 123–135.

Kabat-Zinn, J. (2013). *Full Catastrophe Living*. New York: Bantam Books.

Karatsoreos, I. N., & McEwen, B. S. (2011). Psychobiological allostasis: Resistance, resilience, and vulnerability. *Trends in Cognitive Sciences*, 15(12), 576–584.

Koch, S. C., & Fuchs, T. (2011). Embodied cognition and emotion regulation. *Frontiers in Psychology*, 2, 397.

McEwen, B. S. (2007). Physiology and neurobiology of stress and adaptation. *Physiological Reviews*, 87, 873–904.

Morin, C. M., & Espie, C. A. (2003). *The Oxford Handbook of Sleep and Sleep Disorders*. Oxford University Press.

Porges, S. W. (2011). *The Polyvagal Theory: Neurophysiological Foundations of Emotions, Attachment, Communication, and Self-Regulation*. New York: W. W. Norton.

Rechtschaffen, A., & Kales, A. (1968). *A Manual of Standardized Terminology, Techniques and Scoring System for Sleep Stages of Human Subjects*. UCLA Brain Information Service.

Riemann, D., et al. (2010). The hyperarousal model of insomnia. *Sleep Medicine Reviews*, 14, 19–31.

Sapolsky, R. M. (2004). *Why Zebras Don't Get Ulcers*. New York: Holt Paperbacks.

Sterling, P. (2018). *Allostasis: A Model of Predictive Regulation*. Oxford University Press.

Van Cauter, E., & Knutson, K. L. (2008). Sleep and the epidemic of obesity in children and adults. *European Journal of Endocrinology*, 159(Suppl 1), S59–S66.

Walker, M. P. (2017). *Why We Sleep: Unlocking the Power of Sleep and Dreams*. New York: Scribner.

Yehuda, R. (2015). Neurobiology of PTSD. *Annual Review of Clinical Psychology*, 11, 451–474.

About the Author

Paul Szyarto is the founder of Dreameaz and the creator of the Dreameaz Method™, a systems-based approach to restoring sleep for people who have tried everything and still struggle to rest. His work is shaped not by theory alone, but by lived experience with long-term sleep disruption brought on by sustained stress, responsibility, and nervous system overload.

After decades spent in leadership, entrepreneurship, and advisory roles within high-pressure environments, Paul reached a point where discipline, routines, and conventional advice no longer worked. Sleep did not disappear suddenly. It faded gradually, as it does for many capable, driven people whose systems remain constantly activated. That experience led him away from quick fixes and toward a deeper examination of why sleep breaks down and what actually allows it to return.

Through this process, Paul developed a practical framework that reframes sleep as the outcome of aligned systems rather than a behavior that can be forced. The Dreameaz Method focuses on understanding how daily patterns, biology, emotional load, cognitive intensity, environment, and lifestyle interact to either support or undermine rest. This approach has helped thousands of individuals rebuild predictability, safety, and confidence in their nights.

Paul holds advanced degrees in business, law, and applied artificial intelligence, and brings more than twenty-five years of experience building and leading companies, advising executives, and teaching at the graduate level. Despite these credentials, he does not position himself as a doctor or clinician. His work exists at the intersection of systems thinking, personal recovery, and compassionate realism.

Paul lives in the United States with his family. When he is not writing or developing Dreameaz resources, he continues practicing the same principles he shares with readers, protecting rhythm, honoring recovery, and remembering that sleep is not something to chase, but something to return to.

Learn more about Paul Szyarto at: www.paulszyarto.com

www.ingramcontent.com/pod-product-compliance
Lightning Source LLC
Chambersburg PA
CBHW071448140726
47997CB00005B/1638